BRAIDS AND STYLES FOR LONG HAIR

Written and Edited by

    Andrea Jeffery and Vickie Terner

Drawings: Helen McCallum

Photographer: Roy White

Hair Stylist: Andrea Jeffery

Models: Jennifer Pettigrew
            Andréa Brooks (Parsons)
            Gillian Woolnough

Proofreader: Margaret-Rose Best

Printer: Phoenix Press Inc.

Publisher: Zöpfe 1988

Calgary, Alberta, Canada

ISBN 0-9693543-0-4

This book is affectionately dedicated to the memory of Helen McCallum, our dear friend and professional artist of this book. She spent many hours following the diagrams and instructions which Andrea had prepared.

We appreciate Brian, Sean, Andréa, Frank, Christopher, and Jeffrey for being so patient, understanding, and supportive while we worked on the book.

Thanks also to Margaret-Rose Best (Beauty Culture Teacher for the Calgary Catholic School Board) for the proofreading she did so willingly.

From Roy White, our photographer, we received beautiful shots of our models. His thoughtfulness and humor were free.

Our models deserve a special thanks, as their time was donated on several occasions for the photography.

Vickie & Andrea

Thanks to Vickie for coming up with the idea to write this book, and for all the hours she spent organizing, writing, and working on the computer.

Andrea

Andrea's skill with braiding was the foundation for everything included in this book. She's also a great classroom instructor. Her experience made it possible to specialize in only those methods which were easy for students to learn.

Vickie

PREFACE

My hair has been waist length for many years now, something with which I became very bored in the spring of 1985. Scanning through Continuing Education calendars, my eye caught a class entitled "Get Knotty," offered at the local college. Immediately, I signed up, thinking that braiding had to be better than the same old thing I had been doing.

The first classes got me hooked, and by the end of the session, I had learned enough to know that I wanted to know more. Looking into books at the library and bookstores revealed an almost total absence of material on braiding. The one book I did find was sadly incomplete in terms of what Andrea taught in class.

Long hair is coming back into vogue. I wanted to remember what I had learned in class, and the natural result was a book on braiding; Andrea agreed with enthusiasm.

The book was to be more than just a regular book. It had to show detail of the natural progression of steps involved, not only braiding someone else's hair, but also braiding one's own hair. We wanted to go from simple braids to more difficult ones, again in natural progression. The book also needed to include a variety of ways in which braiding could be combined, adapted, and utilized.

The result is Braids and Styles for Long Hair. It is the accumulation of three years effort for Andrea and I. We know you will like it. Try the braids, and enjoy the results of your own handiwork!

We have used inches rather than centimeters. For metric users one (1) inch equals 2½ centimeters.

The steps presented here are the easiest for students to learn, although in some cases there might be a different method of doing the braid.

Vickie Terner

BRAIDS AND STYLES FOR LONG HAIR

Index

GLOSSARY

Add-on/in: To bring together or join hair from a different area of the head into a strand.

Bangs: A fringe of short hair, generally across the forehead.

Base: The foundation of a section; the section of hair closest to the scalp.

Braid: To weave, interlace, or combine two or more strands together to form a pattern.

Chignon: A knot of hair secured to the head.

Coil: Strands wound or twisted around a center.

Crown: The top of the head, or parietal area of the head.

Cross-over: Outside strand, left or right, comes over middle strand.

Feeding: Adding hair to the braid, from the hairline or nape area.

Figure-of-Eight: Hair twisted into the shape of an eight, horizontally or vertically, on the head.

Fist: All fingers closed and wrapped tightly around a strand of hair.

Flowing Nape: Hair which hangs loose and free at the nape area.

Frontal: The bone which forms the forehead.

Gros-Grain Ribbon: A ribbon with crosswise ribbing.

Hairline: The outline of the scalp, as outlined by the hair around the face.

Horizontal: Runs along or parallel to the horizon. Starting at one temporal area, crossing the occipital bone, and finishing at the opposite temporal area.

Index Finger: Digit next to the thumb.

Intact: As a whole, all together, a single entity.

Invisible: Concealed, out of sight, unable to be seen.

Middle Finger: Digit between the index finger and the ring finger.

Nape:	The back of the head, the base of the hairline.
Occipital:	The bone at the lower back of the head; the bone which forms the back of the skull
One Turn:	Bringing the left outside strand over the middle strand and then right outside strand over middle strand.
Parietal:	The bones which form the sides and top (crown) of the skull.
Pigtail:	A braid made by weaving three strands of hair, without feeding.
Pinch:	The tight grip or squeeze of the thumb and index finger holding a strand of hair.
Plait:	To braid or interweave strands of hair.
Ponytail:	Hair drawn into a single strand or tail.
Roll:	To revolve by turning over and over, generally into a cylindrical shape.
Section:	A sub-division or portion of hair; to divide or separate a portion of hair.
Sphenoid:	A bone above each ear which joins all bones of the skull together.
Strand:	A group of hairs; one of the major parts of a rope or braid.
Temporal:	Bones which form the sides of the head in the ear region (below the parietal bones)
Tension:	Degree of tightness.
Travelling:	Hair that goes from one point to another, according to a predetermined pattern
Vertical:	Upright, lengthwise. In braiding, from the frontal area to the nape area.
Vise:	Clamping or tight grasping of a strand of hair by the index and middle fingers.
Visible:	Can be seen and observed.
Zygomatic:	The bones which form and give shape to the cheeks.

BONES OF THE SKULL

— The following bones will be mentioned throughout this book. The diagram will help you locate the correct area mentioned.

1. Occipital
2. Parietal
3. Frontal
4. Sphenoid
5. Zygomatic
6. Temporal (see both diagrams)
7. Frontal

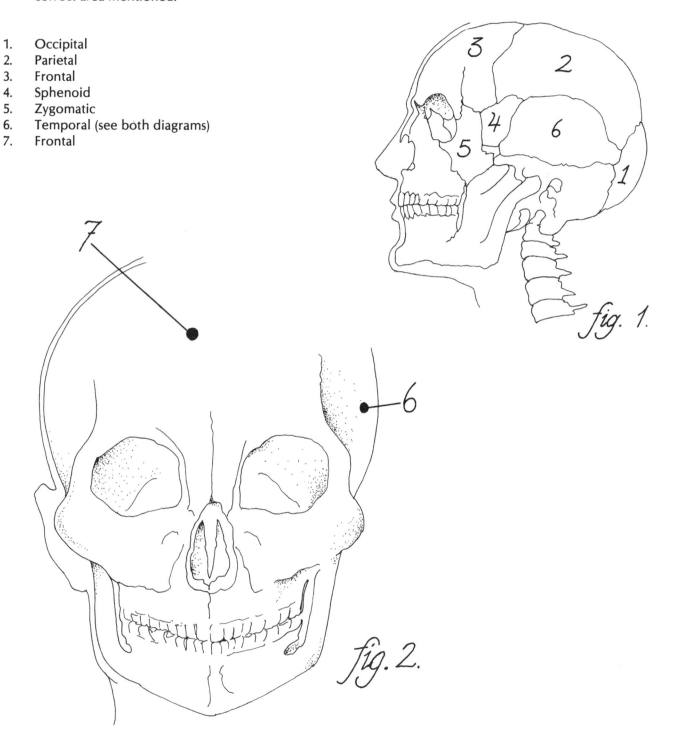

fig. 1.

fig. 2.

HEAD SECTION TERMINOLOGY

The following terms will be used throughout the book. Please familiarize yourself with the terms used for various sections of the head.

1. Crown Area (see both diagrams)
2. Front Center of the hairline
3. Center of the top of the head
4. Top of ear
5. Nape area
6. Base hairline

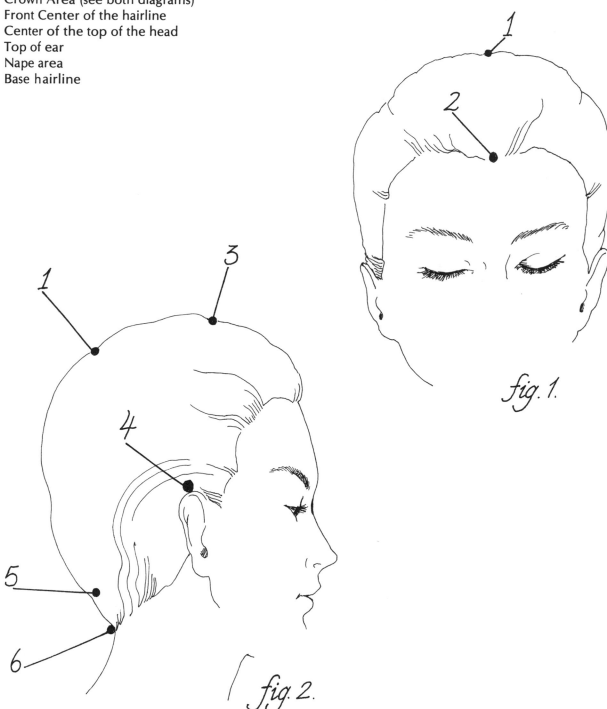

fig. 1.

fig. 2.

FINGERS

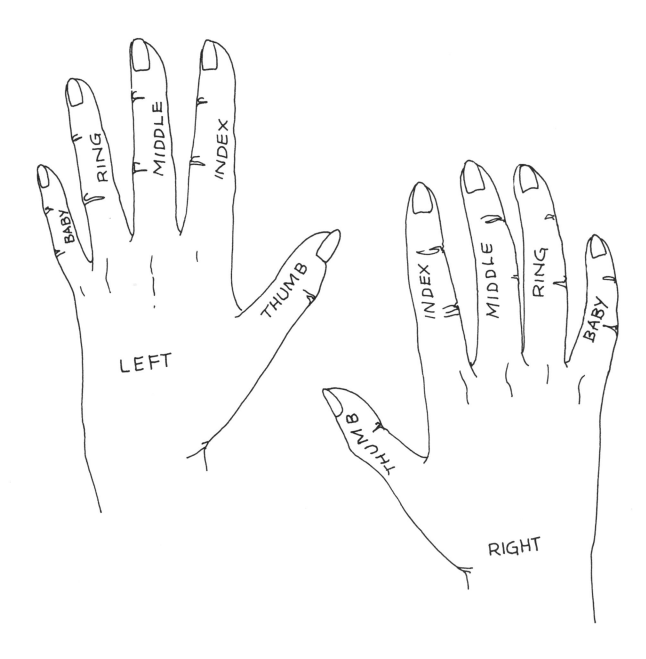

1. *The Beauty of Long Hair*

Throughout history, the beauty of long hair has been recognized by men and women. Women appreciate the feminine qualities it affords them, along with the opportunity to enhance their own appearance. Most men like long hair and find it sexy, both because it is long as well as more flowing and natural.

Long hair has great versatility. It can be worn long and loose, or long and secured in one of many ways. Worn long and loose, it can sweep over a woman's shoulders or down her back. Carefully arranged on the head, it can form a full or partial crown in any one of a dozen different styles.

Long hair can look great for formal occasions - up or down. It's great for informal situations too, - up or down. Partially a matter of preference, long flowing tresses, long loose braids, or hair tied up in a knot or bun - they all have their place for every individual. A bride can look very elegant when her hair is braided around the crown. A veil and flowers fit very naturally around the braid, and the bride looks radiant in a hair style that will be extremely care-free and comfortable all day. Braids keep the head cooler, and hair out of the face, a great asset for sports, windy days, camping trips, as well as some types of work.

Braiding is very easy to do. When correct finger positions are used, strands are in the right place to move exactly where they need to be. Simple styles can be done in ten minutes or less. Even the more complex or time consuming styles can be completed in less than thirty minutes.

Anyone can learn to braid - mothers, fathers, daughters, and even boyfriends. With a few changes in technique, you can even braid your own hair. This is why a separate chapter is included on braiding your own hair. With these basics, anyone can braid their own, or anyone else's hair. And this includes every style demonstrated in this book.

Regardless of age, braids look beautiful. Of course, some variations will look better on children than on others, while others will enhance the features of a mature woman. Often children look prettier and more appealing when their hair is braided with a center part. Braids offer an extensive array in variation of both style and arrangement. While most of our braids are shown adding in all of the hair on the head, great variation can be achieved very simply. For example: braid the hair feeding in just to the back of the ear, basic braid a few turns, then secure with a cloth covered band. This will leave a tail lying down the back of the hair which is left loose. The only limiting factor to the variety of styles that can be done is imagination. Start with the basics, then add more and more steps. And practice!

The only items required for braiding are shoulder length hair (although spot braiding can be done with shorter hair), a brush or comb and fingers.

Hair can be any thickness. Thick hair would be worked in smaller quantities than thin hair, but the result is essentially the same.

Braiding can be done with wet or dry hair, although dry hair is much easier since it slides better. Damp and wet hair are difficult to work with, but tend to produce a tidier, smoother, tighter braid. In either case, it is a matter of preference.

For similar reasons, braiding freshly washed hair is more difficult than hair washed the day before. Freshly shampooed hair is almost too slippery and difficult to work with, whereas day old hair has just enough natural oils to make it fairly easy to braid. Here again, it is personal choice, which practice will help you determine.

And speaking about practice, as with anything else, it's important. At first, the fingers and arms will get tired, but this will soon pass. With practice, skills improve as does the memory in remembering the steps involved. The braids will look better and better, and soon you'll find yourself able to do more and more complex braids.

Practice will help you readily recognize what looks best on different face shapes, as well as where the braid can be adjusted slightly to enhance different features.

Mirrors are not really an advantage when braiding. Try to use them only occasionally to check your work. Usually they tend to create confusion.

Our instructions are generally written for right-handed persons, however, they can easily be used by left-handed persons. Left-handed persons will tend to want to start on the right side of the head, rather than the left as right-handed persons.

Once the hair has been braided, secure with cloth covered bands if a stretch type of closure is to be used. Rubber elastic bands are very hard on the hair and are apt to pull. They also weaken hair strands causing eventual breakage.

2. *Basic Braiding*

Braiding is basically a weaving process where strands of hair are combined to form a pattern. The techniques used for braiding hair are essentially the same as those used when braiding anything else: by taking several sections of hair and crossing them over one another in a definite pattern. As the crossing progresses, plaits of the braid are worked. Each plait is one complete step of the braiding process.

Braiding consists of several steps:

Getting Started — Hand Positions

Working the braid — Plaiting

Tying off — Finishing

The simplest braids begin with 3 strands, and can be worked in two ways: (1) over - the English method, and (2) under - the Dutch method.

The Visible Braid

Hand and Finger Position I

— In making the visible braid, both hands are in similar postitons.

— Instead of only the index finger under the strands, put the index and middle fingers underneath, side by side.

— Right hand: All fingers are under strand #3.

— Left hand: Index and middle finger are under strands #1 and #2.

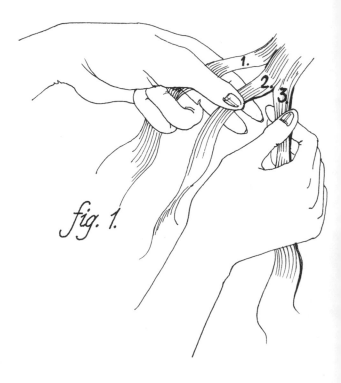

fig. 1.

Hand and Finger Position II

— Place strand #3 between the index and middle fingers.

— <u>Always</u> place the strand so that it lays across the middle finger and under the index finger. (This allows hair to be fed into the 'little vise' easily, without any problems.)

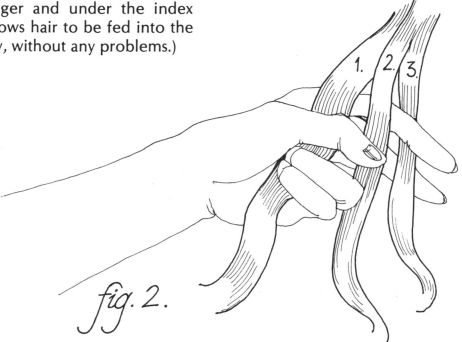

fig. 2.

Visible Braid (No Feeding)

— This is a regular pigtail. Learn this before trying the French Visible Braid with feeding.

— #3 goes under #2.

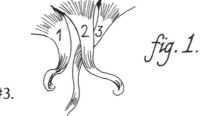

fig. 1.

— #1 goes under strand #3.

— Each outside strand is always put under the strand in the center.

fig. 2.

— #2 goes under #1.

— #3 goes under #2.

— #1 goes under #3.

— #2 goes under #1.

— Repeat this process until the braid is completed.

— Secure with a cloth covered elastic band, 1½ inches from the end of the shaft.

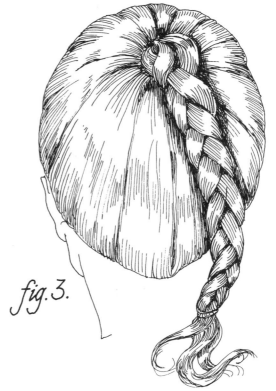

fig. 3.

Helpful Hints

Tension: Tight braiding holds much longer and better than loose braiding. Keep tension consistently tight since braids tend to loosen naturally throughout the day.

Wet or Dry Hair: Braiding can be done with wet or dry hair, generally according to the preference of whoever is doing the braiding. Dry hair tends to slide easier, so is usually not difficult to work with.

Jaw Clips: Place a jaw clip on each strand. Number the jaw clips, going left to right, as the strands in Fig. 1 are numbered. This will make it less complicated to keep track of the strands as braiding progresses.

Invisible Braid

Hand and Finger Position I

— Left Hand - Holds strands #1 and #2.

— Right Hand - Has the outside strand #3, which does the travelling, as shown in the next finger position.

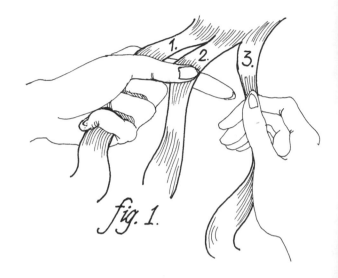

fig. 1.

Hand and Finger Position II

— **Strand #3** - Crosses over strand #2 and is put into the middle finger.

— With the Right Hand, take strand #2 and position the right index finger under strand #3, with right thumb on top of strand #3.

— Correctly done, the right hand position will look like Fig. 3 once strand #1 is brought over into the middle finger of the right hand.

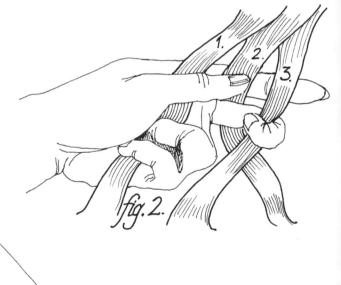

fig. 2.

figure 3.

Invisible Braid (No Feeding)

— This is a regular Pigtail. Learn this before trying the Invisible Braid with feeding.

— #3 goes over #2.

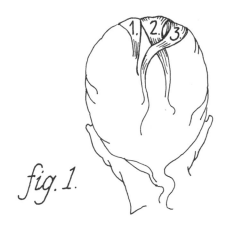

fig. 1.

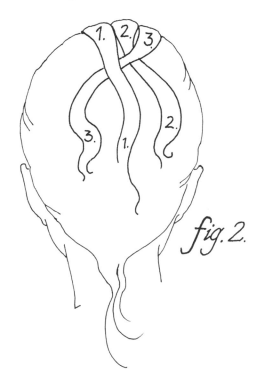

fig. 2.

— #1 goes over #3.

— Notice that each outside strand is always put over the strand in the center.

— #2 strand goes over #1.

— #3 goes over #2.

— #1 goes over #3.

— #2 goes over #1

— Repeat this process until the braid is completed.

— Secure with a cloth covered elastic band, 1½ inches before the end of the shaft.

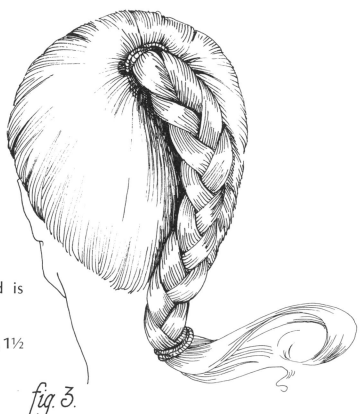

fig. 3.

Helpful Hints

Tension: Care should be taken to maintain moderately tight and consistent tension, creating a tight braid. This will stay secure longer.

Jaw Clips: Place a jaw clip on each strand, then write number one on strand one, number two on strand two, and three on strand three. This will make it much easier to keep track of the strands as braiding progresses.

Finishing: For a cleaner look, bend the tail back under the band after it is twisted around the hair for the last time.

Ribbon or lace can be added, either tied over the elastic, or woven through the braid.

The braid itself can be handled in several different ways. In addition to being left loose, it can be twisted and pinned into a coil or chignon, or secured under the beginning of the braid itself.

3. *Intermediate Braiding*

THE FRENCH BRAID - VISIBLE

— Divide the section into three equal strands.

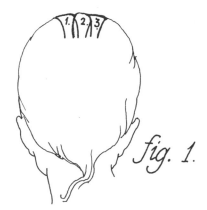

fig. 1.

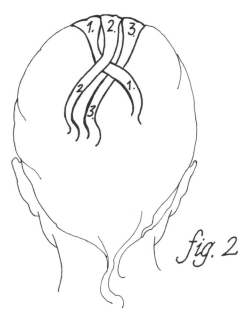

fig. 2

— Cross strand #1 under strand #2.

— Now take strand #3 under strand #1.

— Adjust to maintain tight tension.

— Feed section 'A' into strand #2 and with this cross under strand #3.

— Feed section 'B' into strand #1 and cross this under strand #2A.

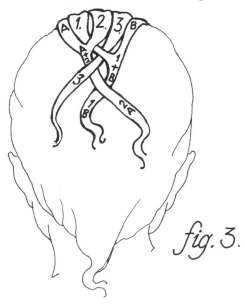

fig. 3.

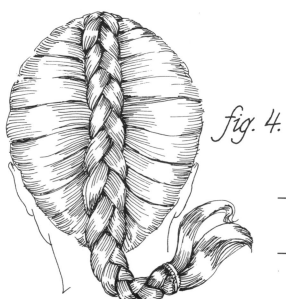

fig. 4.

— Continue, repeating the steps in Figure 3 until all hair has been added in.

— Finish braiding to the end of the hair using the Basic Braid (as in Figure 2).

Helpful Hints

Hand Positions: Correct hand positions helps to keep tension consistent and tight. One hand serves as a holding mechanism for maintaining constant tension as braiding proceeds, which leaves the other hand free to work the braid.

Tension: Working hands should lie almost on the scalp as the braiding progresses. Always hold the strands close together, firmly in place, to maintain a smooth tight braid.

Stance: Always keep the section you're braiding in front of your body, as your hands will set up the direction of the braid. Determine the direction the braid will proceed before beginning your braid.

Sectioning: Small sections generally result in a nicer looking braid, and are easier to work with once the braider is skilled. For practice purposes use larger sections.

When adding a new section, take all hair from the hairline to the braid and add it into the catcher finger. Smooth it with the working fingers so that all hairs in the section lay flat upon the head.

Bangs: Bangs can be worked into the braid if they are long enough, otherwise, start the braid just behind the bangs.

THE FRENCH BRAID - INVISIBLE

— Divide the section into three equal strands.

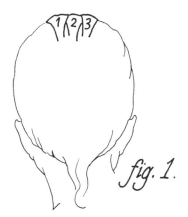

fig. 1.

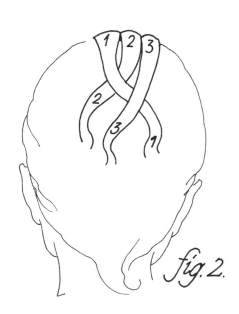

fig. 2.

— Cross strand #1 over strand #2.

— Take strand #3 over strand #1.

— Adjust to maintain tight tension.

— Feed section 'A' to strand #2, then cross combined strand over strand #3.

— Feed section 'B' to strand #1 and cross over strand #2A.

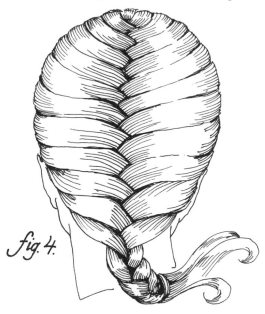

fig. 4.

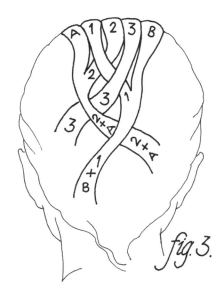

fig. 3.

— Continue, repeating the steps in Figure 3 until all hair has been added in.

— Finish braiding using only strands #1, #2, #3 as in Figure 2.

— Figure 4 is a completed Invisible French Braid.

Helpful Hints

Hand Positions: Proper hand position helps to keep tension consistent and tight. Braid with the palms up in order to clearly see movement of the strands.

The hand position serves a dual purpose: (1) one hand serves as a holding mechanism for maintaining constant tension as the braiding proceeds, and (2) it leaves the other hand free to work.

Tension: As braiding continues, both hands should lie on the scalp, palms up, the strands close together, firmly in place. Braids tend to loosen naturally, hence moderately tight tension should be maintained.

Stance: Braids should move directly toward the braider. Before starting, determine where the braid should start and end. Stand directly behind the working area. Your hands set up the direction of the braid, but the head area at which you stand will determine in what area your braid will end.

Starting Section Shapes: Starting sections can be taken in a rectangular or triangular shape. The triangle, taken in a 1 - 1½" length, has its section added on at roughly 45 degree angles. This tends to produce a slightly looser and less durable braid. The rectangle, taken about 2" by 1", has sections added in almost straight up, making it slightly more durable.

Sectioning: Small sections generally result in a nicer looking braid, and are easier to work with once the braider is skilled. For practice purposes, use larger sections.

Feeding the strands requires that all hair from the hairline to the braid is added into the catcher finger. Smoothing means that all hair in the section lays flat upon the head.

Bangs: Work bangs into the braid if they are long enough, otherwise start the braid just behind the bangs.

Finishing: Hair that is braided to the end can be left hanging, or secured underneath the nape plaits. This can be done because the Invisible Braid creates a tunnel underneath the braid into which the tail can be tucked.

Variations: This braid can be worked high as in a plait around the crown of the head, or lower down at any of several different places. Included here would be halfway down the head just above the ears, or along the hairline. Primarily a matter of preference, lie of the braid can be determined by how formal or informal a style is desired, as well as what looks best.

THE MODIFIED FRENCH BRAID

The French Braid can be modified slightly so instead of adding in from two sides, hair is added in from only one side. The result is a much smoother area above the braid.

This method is best worked with a part, at the center or on the side. It can be worked with the Visible or Invisible Braid, however, the result is much prettier and more obvious when the Invisible method is used.

Modified Invisible

Use the same hand positions as for the Invisible French Braid.

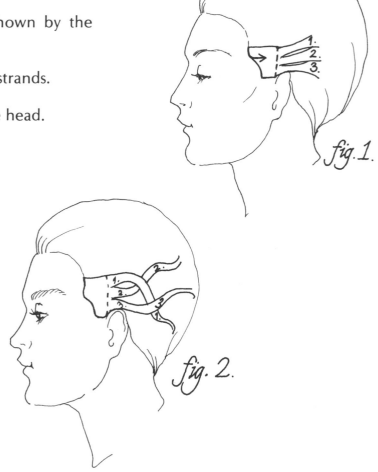

— Take a section of hair, as shown by the dashes.

— Divide the section into three strands.

— Work horizontally around the head.

fig. 1.

— #1 strand goes over #2.

— #3 strand goes over #1.

fig. 2.

- Feed only from the bottom, as shown by 'A' in Figure 1.

- #1 goes over #2.

- #3 goes over #1.

- #2 goes over #3.

- #1A goes over #2.

- #3A goes over #1A.

- #2A goes over #3A.

- #1A goes over #2A.

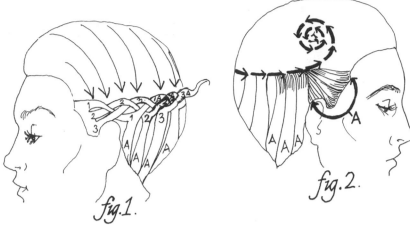

fig.1. fig.2.

- Continue in this manner around the head. All top hair comes under the braid, and is then added in. Arrows show the hair coming from the center part in Figure 1.

- When the braid reaches the back of the opposite ear, direct all hair at the temple area back as one strand. Feed it into the braid.

- Arrows show the direction in which to coil the end of the finished braid.

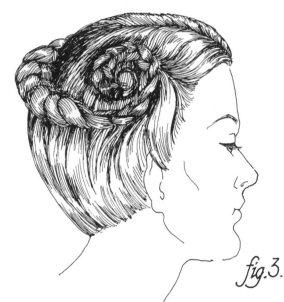

fig.3.

Helpful Hints

Line: Braids can lie along several different 'lines' upon the head: (1) starting at the forehead going around the crown and returning to the forehead, (2) from the forehead to a point halfway between the back of the crown and the nape, (3) along the hairline to the nape of the neck, as well as from one temple to the other.

Stance: Determine where the braid will lie before starting. Keep the working area directly in front of you, so that your hands can properly set up the direction of the braid.

Right Handed/Left Handed Start: For better control of the hair, right handed braiders should start on the left side of the head, and left handed braiders on the right.

4. *Self Braiding*

THE VISIBLE BRAID

The following terminology saves repetition of all the finger positions. It also makes understanding the process of braiding easier to comprehend.

Vise: Middle finger and index finger holding a strand of hair.
Pinch: Thumb and index finger holding a strand of hair.
Fist: All fingers of one hand around a strand. Ring finger and baby finger remain around strand after other fingers leave.

This braid does not have head diagrams, as you will be doing it on yourself, rather, instructions only. Use the proper hand positions that are suggested as follows:

Finger and Hand Position I

— When braiding one's own hair, the hands are always palms down.

— Divide the section of hair into three strands.

— Left Hand: Strand #1 (left outside strand) goes into the ring finger and baby finger. The end of strand #1 will hang over the thumb.

— Strand #2 (middle strand) goes between the index and middle fingers.

— Strand #3 is held by the right hand.

Finger and Hand Position II

— Place strand #3 between the thumb and index finger.

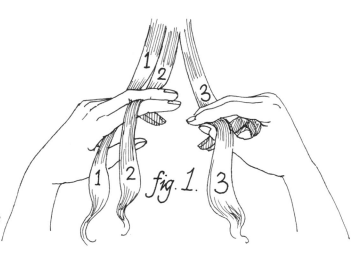

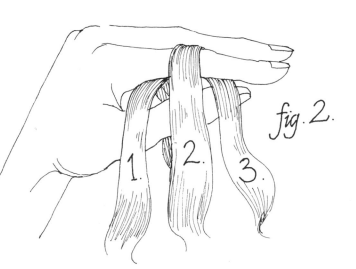

Working the Braid

— Left Hand: Fist outside strand. Put middle strand in vise. Pinch outside strand (right strand).

— Right Hand: Fist what is in left vise. Put strand from left pinched area into right vise. Strand from left fist goes into right pinch.

— Left Hand: Fist what is in right vise. Vise what is in right pinch. Pinch what is in right fist. Now feed hair into what you have just pinched.

— Right Hand: Fist what is in left vise. Vise what is pinched in left hand. Pinch what is fisted in left hand. Now feed into what you just pinched.

— Repeat this procedure until all feeding into the braid is completed.

— Continue with braiding the pigtail (right under and left under).

— Fasten with and elastic.

THE INVISIBLE BRAID

The use of a few basic terms saves repetition of the finger positions. It also makes the braiding process easier to understand. The terms, and their meaning for Invisible Braiding, follow.

Fist: All four fingers around a strand of hair.
Pinch: Thumb and index finger holding a strand of hair.
Feeder: The feeder finger is the middle finger which catches hair when it is fed into the braid. The hair is placed between the middle finger and the index finger.

No head diagrams are included for this braid, as you will be doing it on yourself. Use the proper hand positions, suggested below.

Finger and Hand Position I

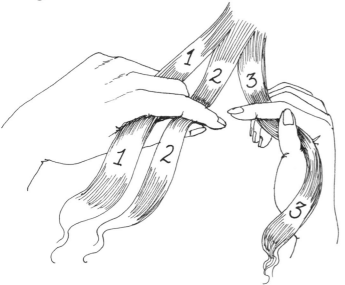

— When braiding one's own hair, the hands are always palms down.

— Divide the section of hair into three strands.

— Left Hand: Strand #1 (the left outside strand) goes into the ring finger and baby finger. The end of strand #1 will hang over the thumb.

— Strand #2 (middle strand) goes between the index finger and thumb.

— Strand #3 is held by the right hand.

Finger and Hand Position II

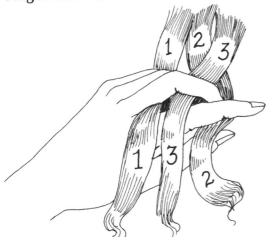

— Place strand #3 into the middle finger.

— Left Hand: Fist the left outside strand. Pinch the middle strand. Cross the right outside strand into the middle finger.

— Right Hand: Fist what is pinched in left hand. Pinch what is in the feeder finger. Cross the left outside strand into the feeder finger.

— Left Hand: Fist what is pinched in the right hand. Pinch what is in the feeder finger. Cross the right outside strand into the left feeder finger.

— Pick up a new section of hair and feed it into the left feeder finger.

— Right Hand: Fist what was pinched in the left hand. Pinch what is in the feeder finger. Cross the left outside strand into the right feeder finger.

— Use left hand to pick up a new section of hair and feed it into the right feeder finger.

— Repeat this procedure until you run out of hair to feed in. Continue the braid, using only the three strands until two inches before the end of the hair shaft. Tie off with an elastic.

— Remember: Fist
                Pinch
                Cross over

THE MODIFIED METHOD

The terms, and their meanings, for the modified braid are:

Fist: All four fingers around a strand of hair.
Pinch: Thumb and index finger holding a strand of hair.
Feeder Finger: The middle finger which catches hair.

Use the Invisible braid method, but only feed from the bottom (hairline). The top strand never gets fed, but crosses over to the middle.

— Make a rectangular section as shown by the broken lines.

— Divide the section into three strands.

— Work horizontally around the head.

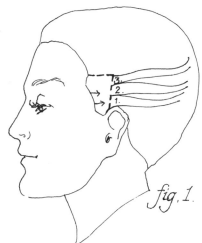

fig. 1.

Arm & Hand Position

— Use the self-braid hand position.

— The left elbow should be raised and pointing outward.

— The right arm should be raised and over the top of the head.

— As you reach the center back of the head, your arm position will resemble Figure 2.

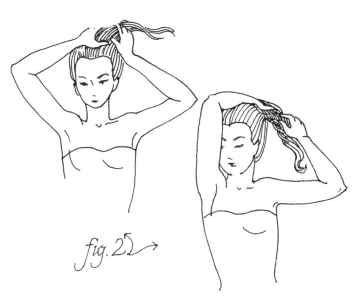

fig. 2.

Working the Braid

— Right Hand: Fist the top strand (#3). Pinch the middle strand (#2). Cross the bottom strand (#1) over the middle strand (#2).

— Left Hand: Fist what is pinched in the right hand. Pinch what is in the right feeder finger. Cross what's in the right fist into the left feeder finger.

— Right Hand: Fist what is pinched in the left hand. Pinch what is in the left feeder finger. Cross what is in the left hand into the right feeder finger. Pick up a section of hair from the hairline and feed it into the right feeder finger.

— Left Hand: Fist what is pinched in the right hand. Pinch what is in the right feeder finger. Cross what is in the right fist into the left feeder finger. DO NOT FEED!

— *Right Hand: Fist what is pinched in the left hand. Pinch what is in the left feeder finger. Cross what is in the left fist into the right feeder finger. Pick up a section of hair from the hairline and feed into the right feeder finger.

— *Left Hand: Fist what is pinched in the right hand. Pinch what is in the right feeder finger. Cross what is in the right fist into the left feeder finger. DO NOT FEED.

— Repeat *Right Hand and *Left Hand until braid is completed.

— Remember: Fist
　　　　　Pinch
　　　　　Cross over

THE TWO STRAND

The following terms save constant repetition of the finger positions, while at the same time making the braiding process easier to comprehend.

Feeder Finger: The middle finger.
Pincher: The index finger and thumb holding a strand of hair.

This braid has diagrams for the hand positions, with instructions only for the braiding process. Use the correct hand positions, as follows.

Finger and Hand Position I

— When braiding your own hair, the hands are always palms down.

— Divide the hair into two sections.

— Left Hand: Fist strand #1. Cross strand #2 into feeder finger.

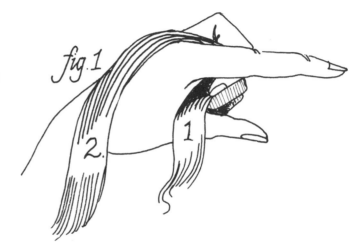

fig.1

Finger and Hand Position II

— Right Hand: Fist what is in the left hand fist (#1). Pinch what is in the left hand feeder finger (#2). Feed hair into the right feeder finger (F).

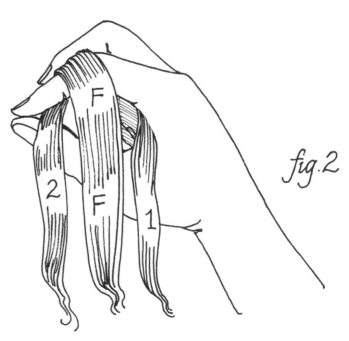

fig.2

25

— Left Hand: Fist what is pinched in the right hand. Pinch what is in the feeder finger of the right hand, as well as what you've fisted in the right hand. (The two become one strand and are held together.)

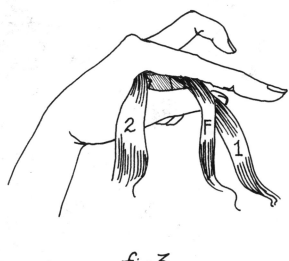

fig.3.

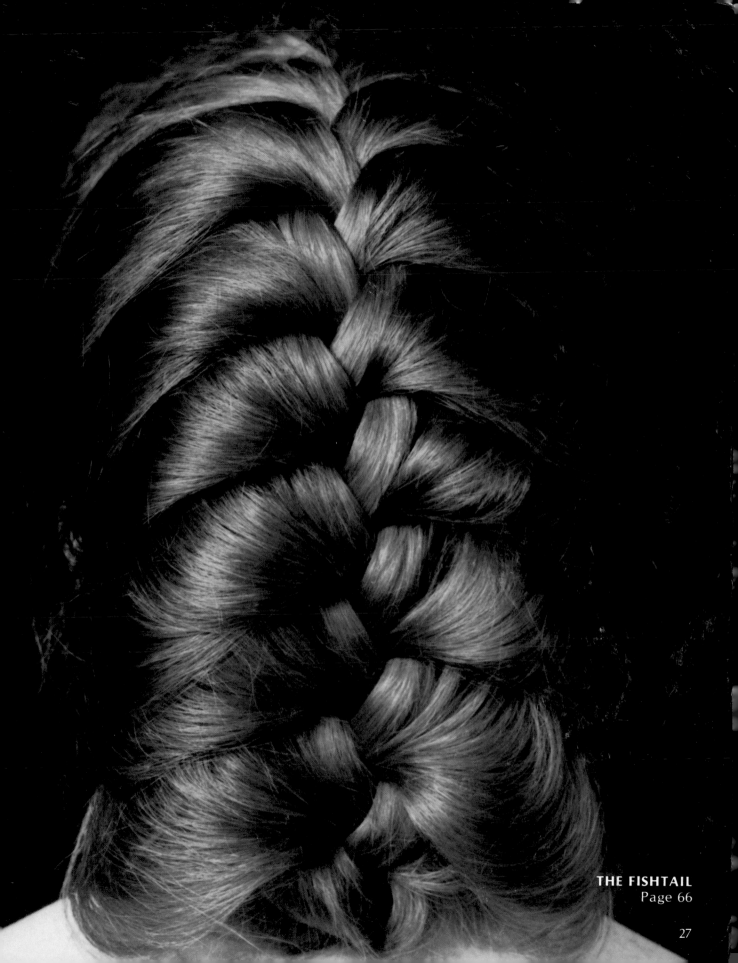

THE FISHTAIL
Page 66

27

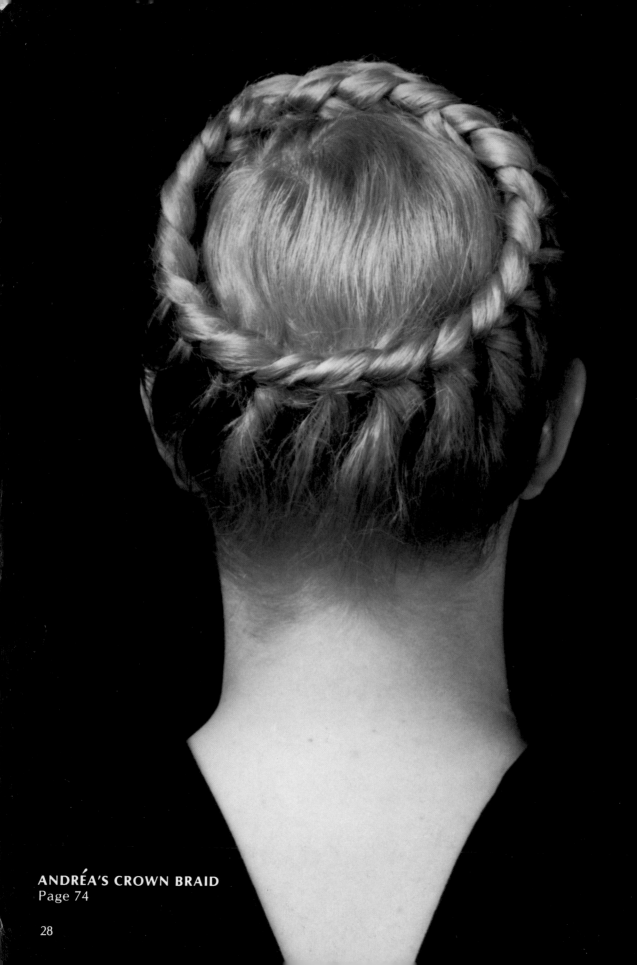

ANDRÉA'S CROWN BRAID
Page 74

28

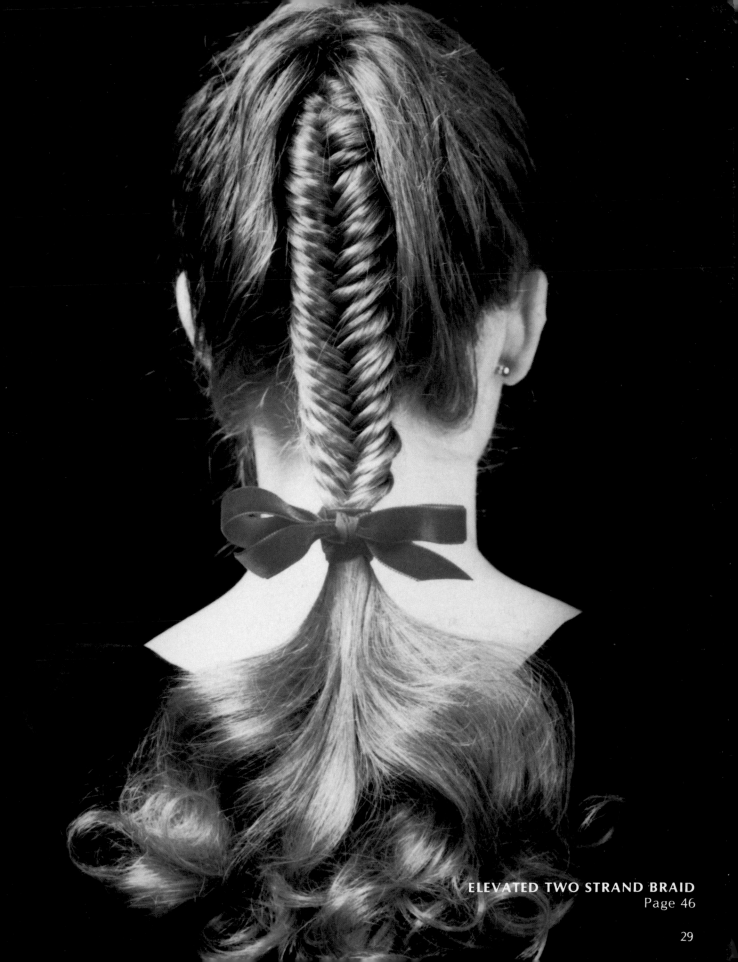

ELEVATED TWO STRAND BRAID
Page 46

29

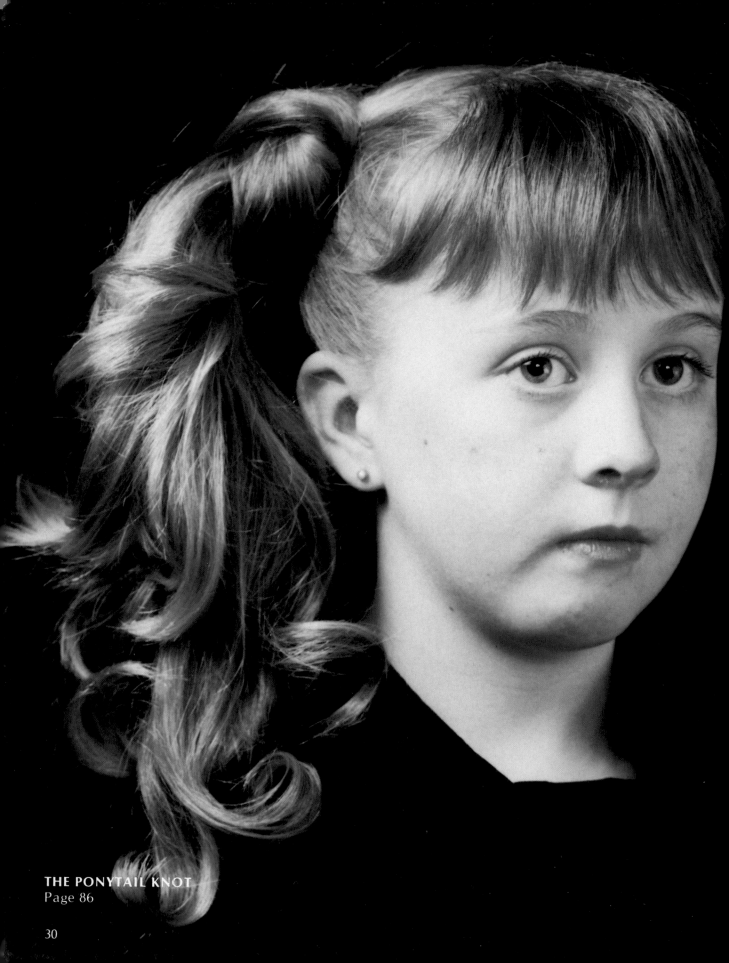

THE PONYTAIL KNOT
Page 86

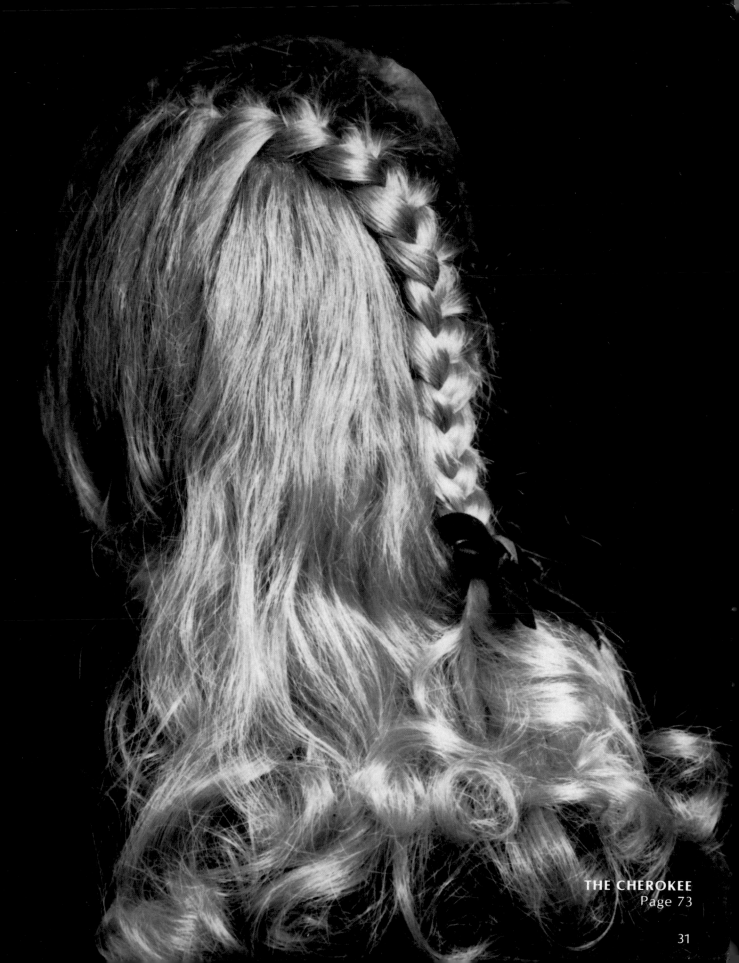

THE CHEROKEE
Page 73

31

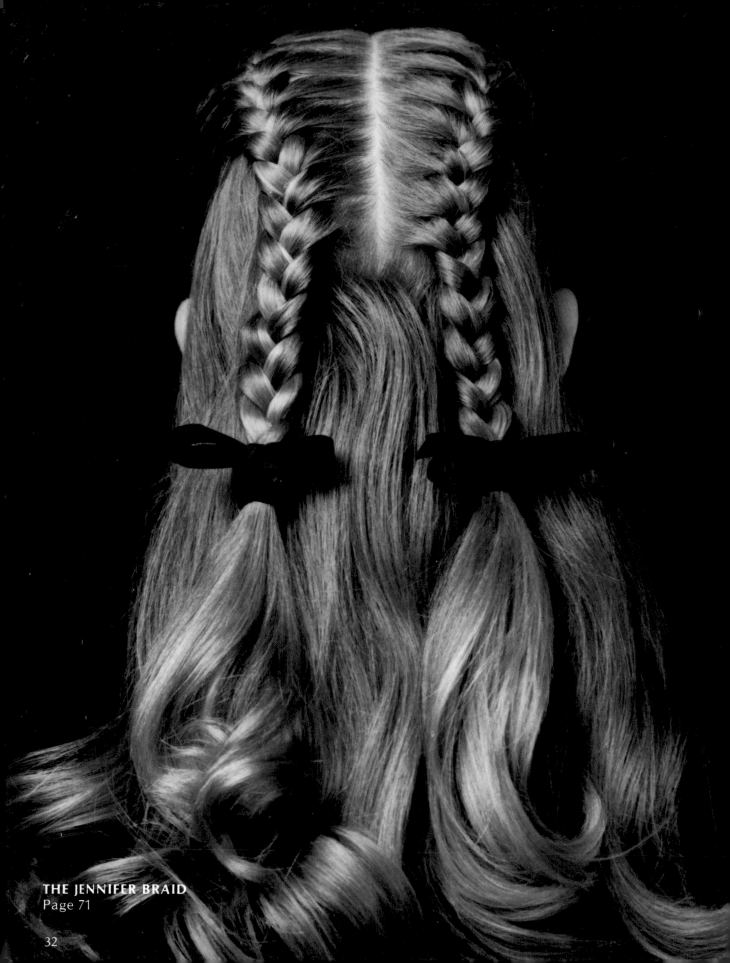

THE JENNIFER BRAID
Page 71

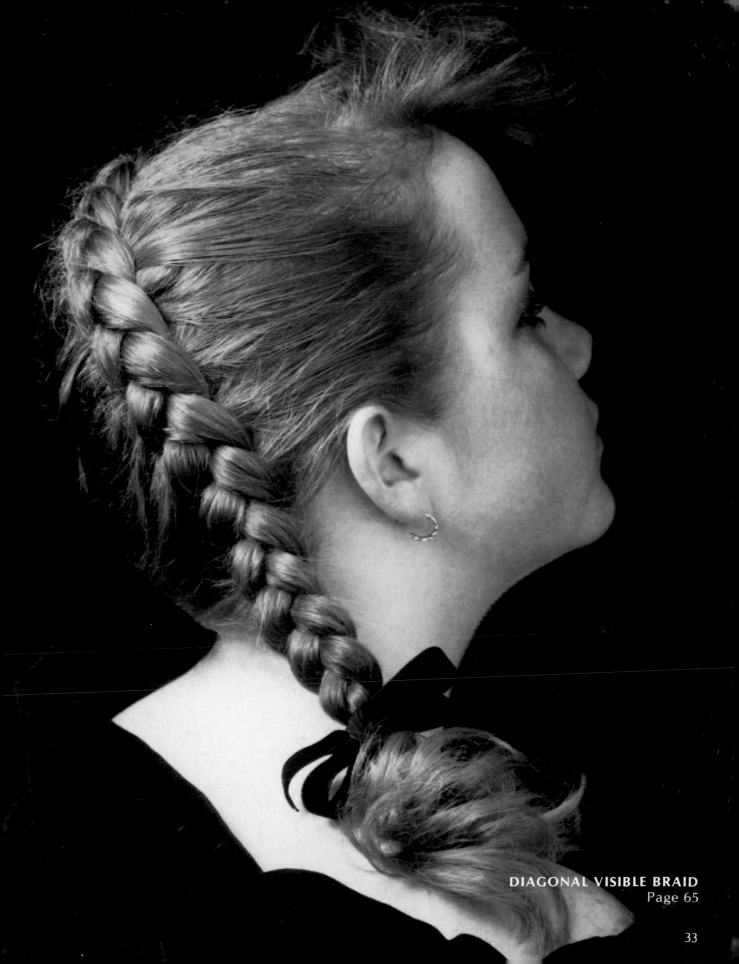

DIAGONAL VISIBLE BRAID
Page 65

33

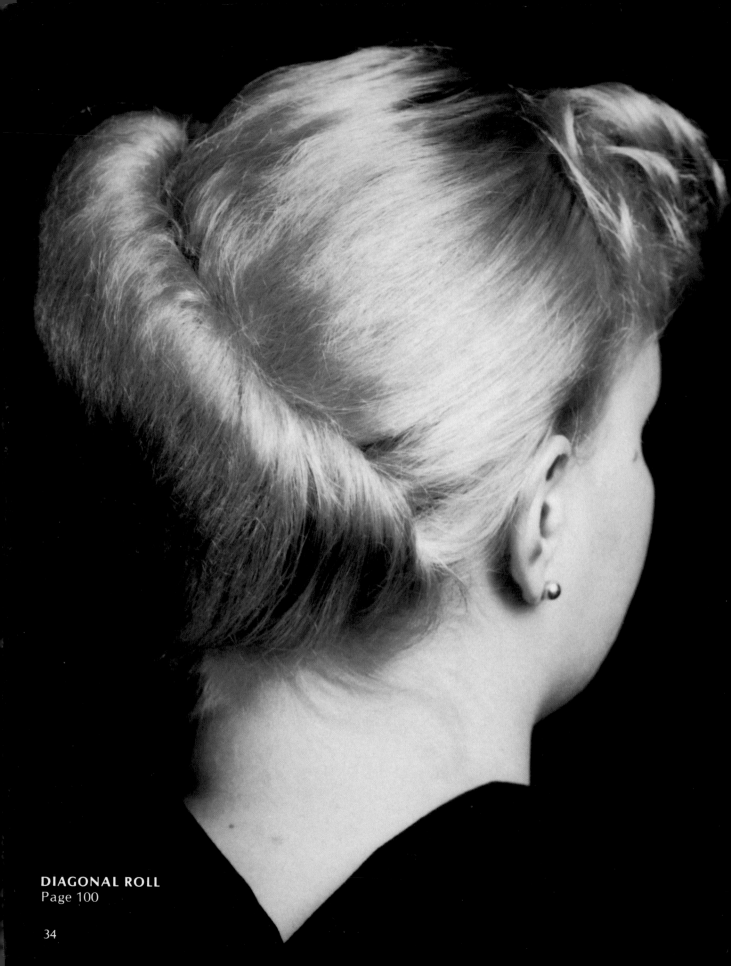

DIAGONAL ROLL
Page 100

34

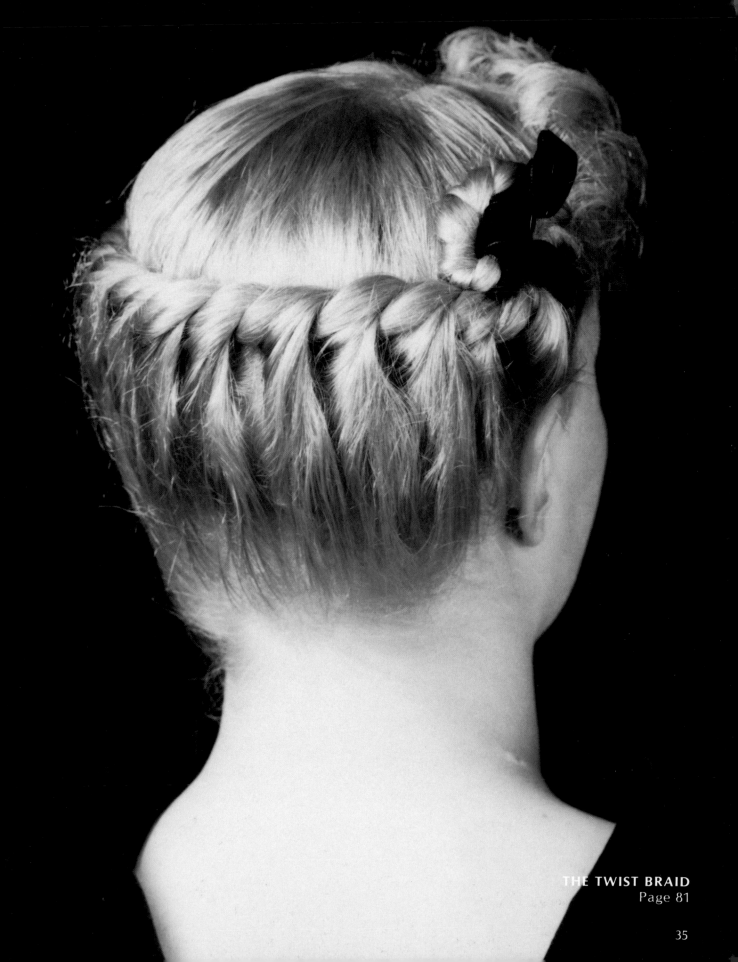

THE TWIST BRAID
Page 81

35

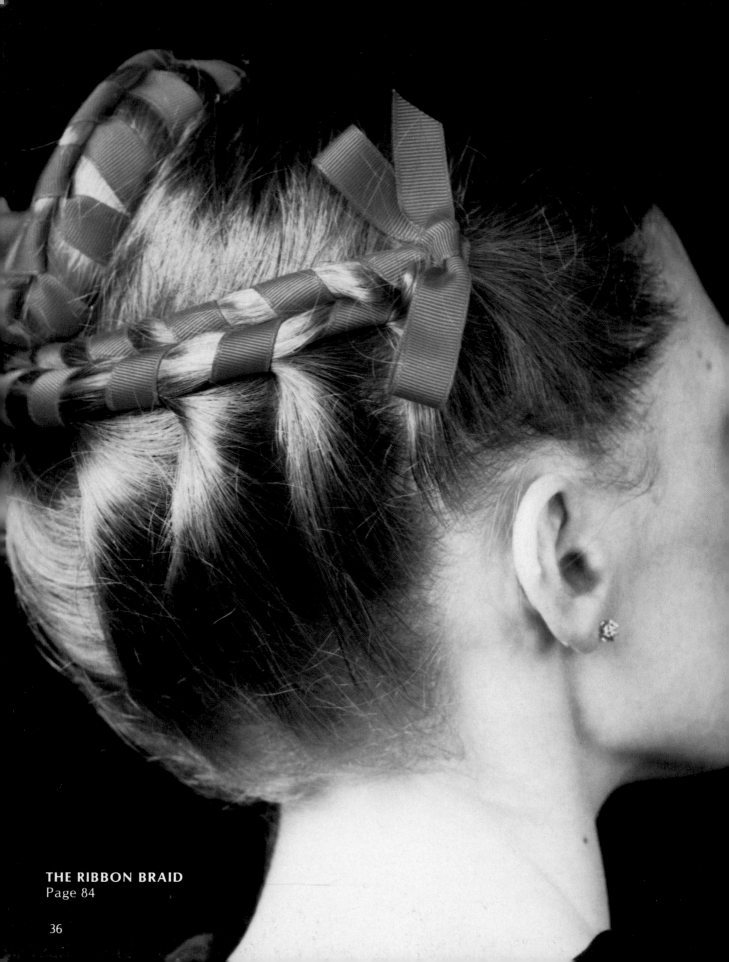

THE RIBBON BRAID
Page 84

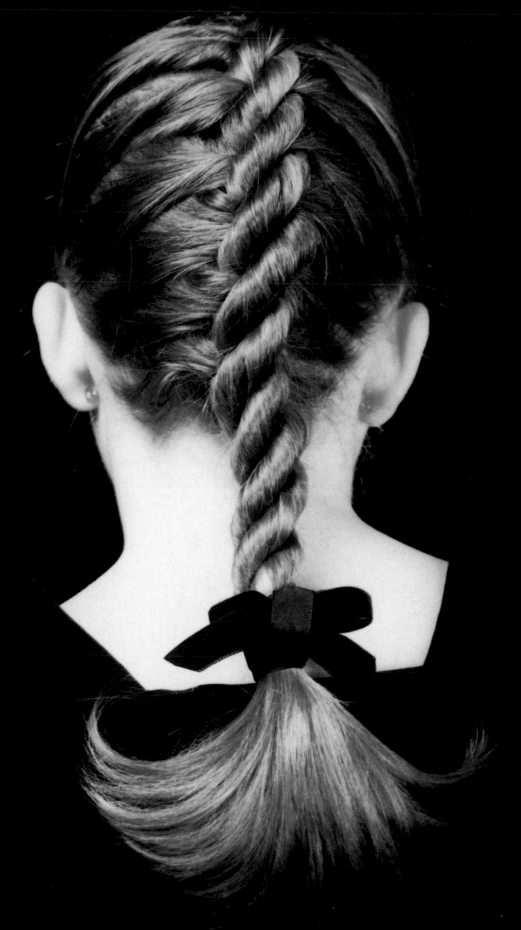

THE ROPE
Page 49

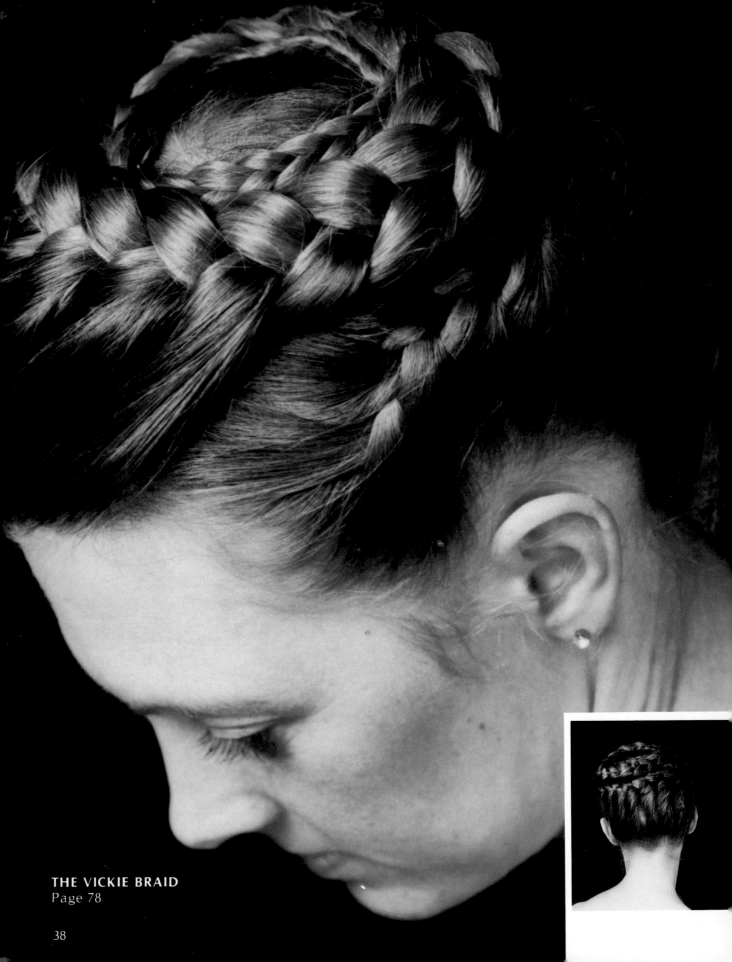

THE VICKIE BRAID
Page 78

5. *Advanced Braiding*

TWO STRAND PONYTAIL

— Brush the hair into a ponytail.

— Divide the hair into two strands.

Finger and Hand Position I

— Bring strand #1 across the top of strand #2.

— Have the left index finger under strand #2, with the thumb on strand #1, as in Figure 1.

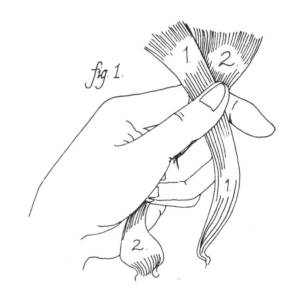

Finger and Hand Position II

— Take a feed section ('F') from strand #2 (the right side), and place it into all three fingers (baby, ring, and middle) of the left hand.

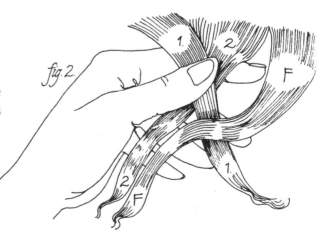

Working the Braid

— Brush the hair into a pony tail.

— Divide the hair into two strands.

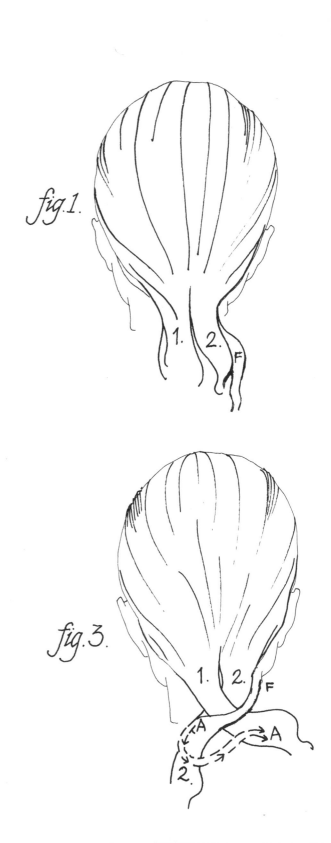

fig.1.

— Take a feed ('F') section from strand #2. Cross 'F' over strand #1 and join it up with strand #2.

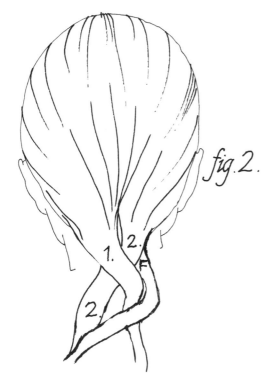

fig.2.

— Take a fine strand of hair, 'A' from the outside of strand #2. (The broken line shows where and what thickness to take.)

fig.3.

40

— 'A' crosses over the rest of #2, and goes over to #1, joining up with #1.

— Do the same thing with 'B', taking it across #1 so that it joins up with #2.

— Repeat these steps until the braid is two inches from the end of the hair shaft.

— Tie off the braid with an elastic.

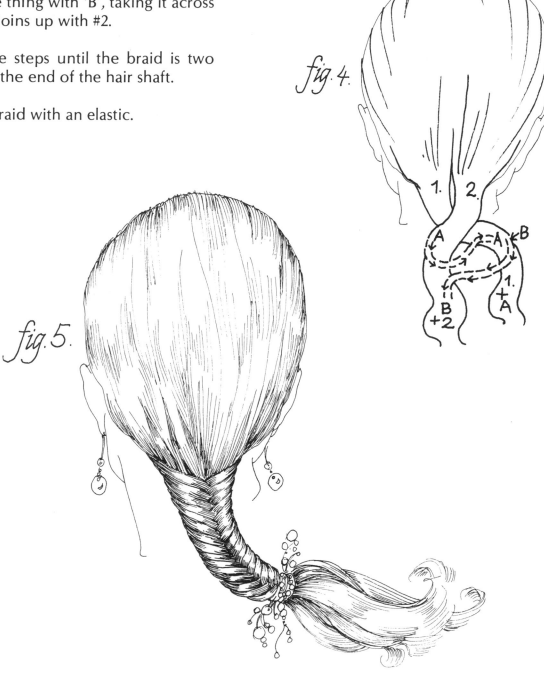

fig. 4.

fig. 5.

TWO STRAND BRAID

— Divide the first section into two strands.

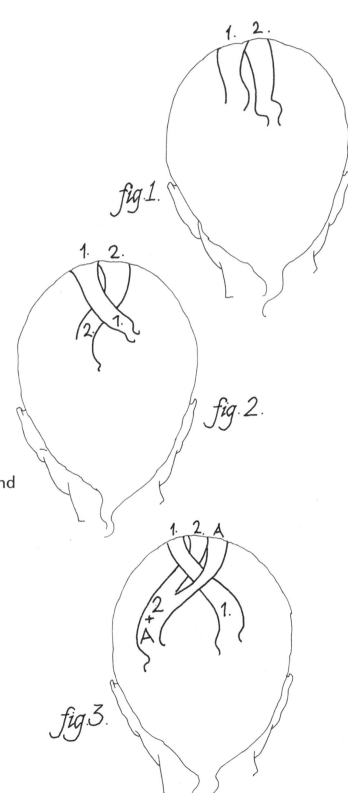

fig.1.

— Cross strand #1 over strand #2.

fig.2.

— From the right, feed strand 'A' into strand #2.

— Strand #2 and 'A' become one strand.

— Now you have two strands again.

fig.3.

— Cross 'B' over #2 + 'A' and join it up with
strand #1.

— Repeat Figure 3 and Figure 4 until all hair
has been fed into the braid.

— You will end up with two thick strands, as
shown in Figure 5.

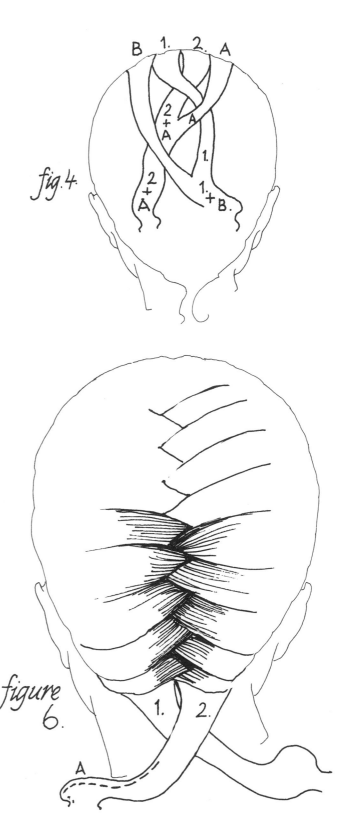

fig. 4.

— Finish the tail by braiding to the end as you
would for a two strand ponytail.

— Take a fine section, 'A' from the outside of
strand #2. (The dotted line shows where and
what thickness to take.)

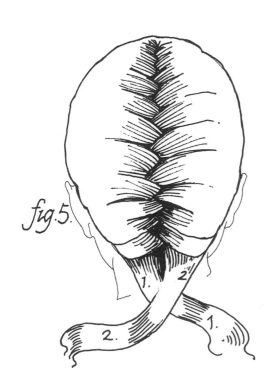

fig. 5.

figure 6.

— 'A' (one-quarter of strand #2) crosses over the remainder of strand #2, and on over to #1, joining up with #1.

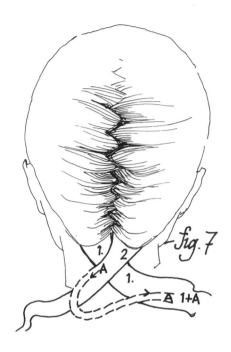

fig. 7

— The same thing is done with 'B'. 'B' goes across #1, to join up with strand #2. Repeat until the braid is completed.

— Tie off the end with an elastic.

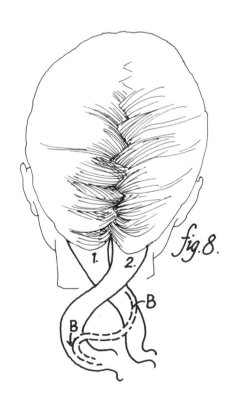

fig. 8.

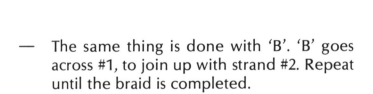

44

— Figure 9 shows the completed Two Strand
  Braid.

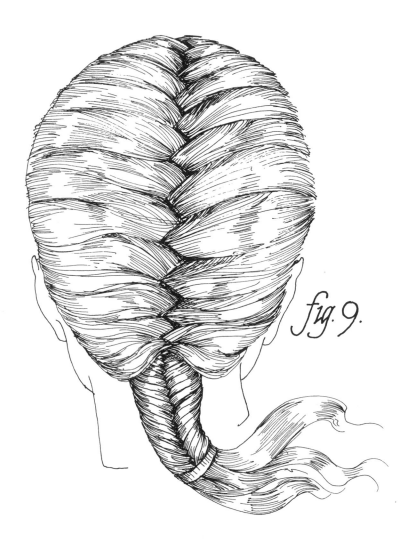

fig. 9.

Helpful Hints

Tension: It is very important to maintain tight tension when doing the Two Strand Braid.

ELEVATED TWO STRAND BRAID

— Start the Elevated Two Strand Braid using the same method as the Two Strand Braid.

— When the crown area is reached ('C'), bring the feeding strands up to 'C'. The hand that is holding the braid, thus keeping tight tension, should rest on the crown.

— Continue braiding until all hair is fed into the braid.

— Proceed to braid the pigtail using the Two Strand Braid method.

— Secure the pigtail with an elastic once the braid is completed.

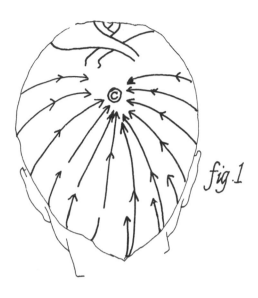

fig.1

— Figure 3 illustrates a finished Elevated Two Strand Braid.

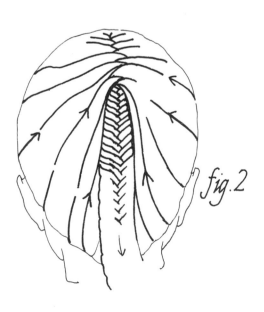

fig.2

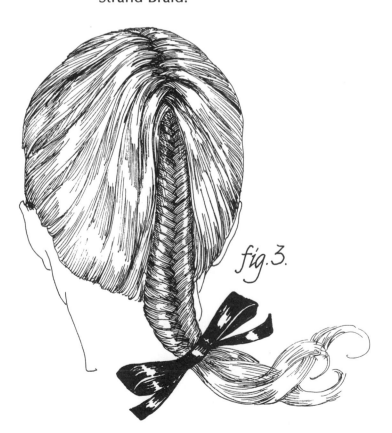

fig.3.

ROPE PIGTAIL

— Make one ponytail of all of the hair.

— Section 'A': Start the rope like an Invisible Braid by taking #3 over #2, and #1 over #3.

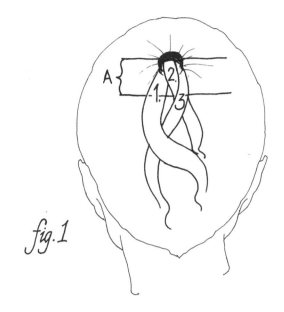

fig.1

— In Figure 2, the letters symbolize the following:
  'R' = Right
  'M' = Middle
  'L' = Left

— Section 'B': Twist 'R' strand 3 or 4 times clockwise.

— Strand 'R' goes over strand 'M'.

— Twist 'L' strand and take it under 'R' strand.

— Section 'C': Twist 'R' and take it over 'M' ('R' becomes 'M'.)

— Twist 'L' and put it under 'M' ('M' becomes 'L').

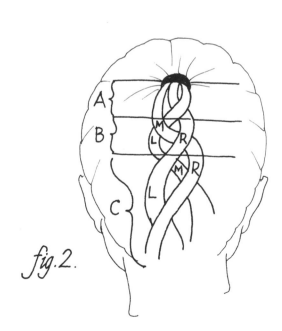

fig.2.

— The right strand always goes over, the left always under. Always twist the strands clockwise.

— If one strand is twisted the wrong way (counter-clockwise), the finished rope will come undone after being tied off.

— Complete the Rope Pigtail.

— Secure tightly with an elastic.

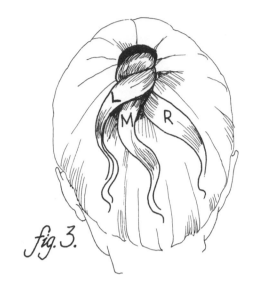

fig. 3.

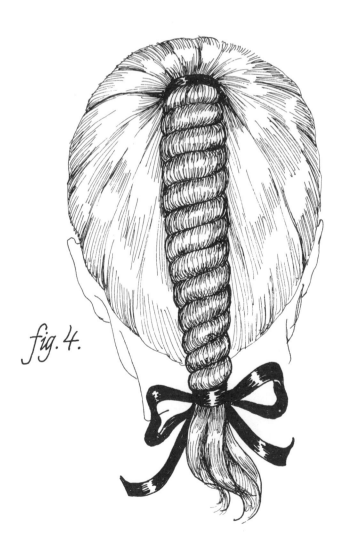

fig. 4.

THE ROPE

— Cross #3 over #2.

— Cross #1 over #3.

— After each strand is fed, twist it to the right two or three times.

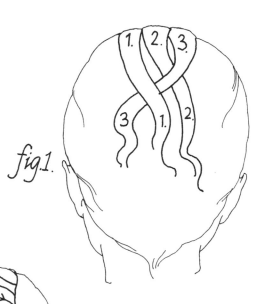

fig.1.

— Feed #2 (It becomes 2A).

— #2A goes over #1.

— Feed #3 (It becomes #3B).

— #3B goes under #2A.

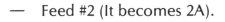

fig.2.

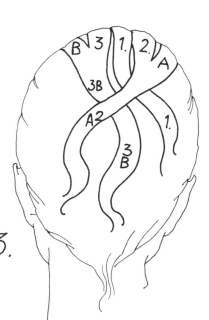

fig 3.

- #1 is fed from 'A' side.

- #1A crosses over #3B.

- #2 is fed again, and then goes under #1A. Notice that the numbers 1, 2, and 3 change from 'A' to 'B' because of their positioning (left, right, left).

- #3 is fed again and crosses over #2.

- #1 is fed again and goes under #3.

- #2 is fed again and goes over #1.

- The strands on the right side always go over.

- Strands on the left side always go under.

- Twisting is always to the right.

- When the rope is finished, tie it off with an elastic.

- If the rope unravels, then twisting was not consistent to the right.

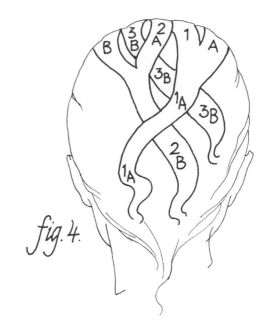

fig. 4.

- Figure 5 shows the rope after feeding is finished.

- To complete, continue twisting and braiding, as before.

- Twist 'C' two or three times to the right and bring it over 'B'.

- Twist 'A' and take it under 'C' ('C' is in the middle at this point).

- Continue until near the end, then fasten with an elastic.

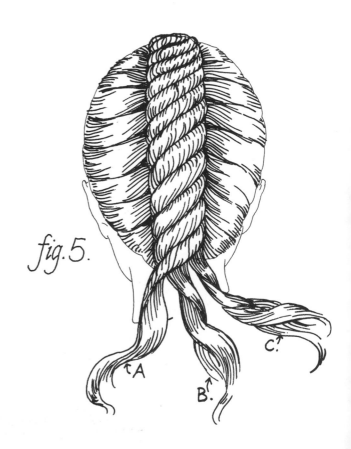

fig. 5.

— Figure 6 is a side view of the rope.

— Figure 7 is a back view of the completed rope.

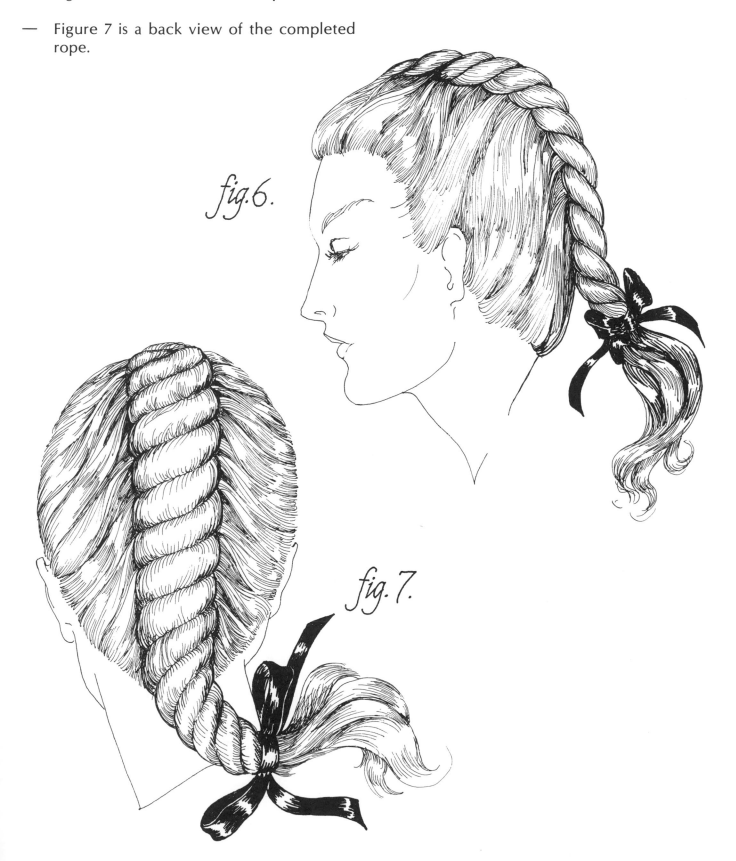

fig. 6.

fig. 7.

FOUR STRAND PONYTAIL

— Figure 1 shows how to separate the ponytail into four strands.

— #4 strand crosses over #3 and goes under #2.

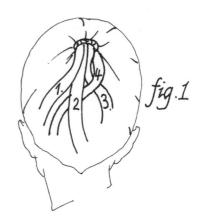

fig.1

— Take #1 strand and go under #4.

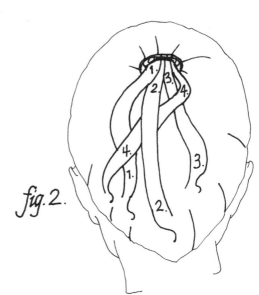

fig.2.

— The outside right strand is #3, so #3 crosses over #2 and then under #1.

— The left outside strand is now #4, so #4 goes under #3.

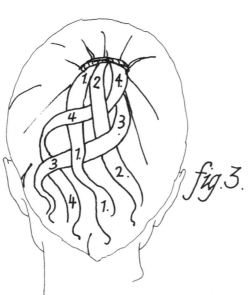

fig.3.

- Continue braiding using the method as follows:

- Right outside strand (strand closest to the right ear) always goes OVER the strand next to it and then UNDER the following strand.

- The left outside strand (strand closest to the left ear) only goes UNDER the strand next to it.

- Consequently, the resulting pattern is the right outside strand goes over and under, and the left outside strand goes under.

- Continue this pattern until two inches before the end of the shaft.

- Tie off with an elastic.

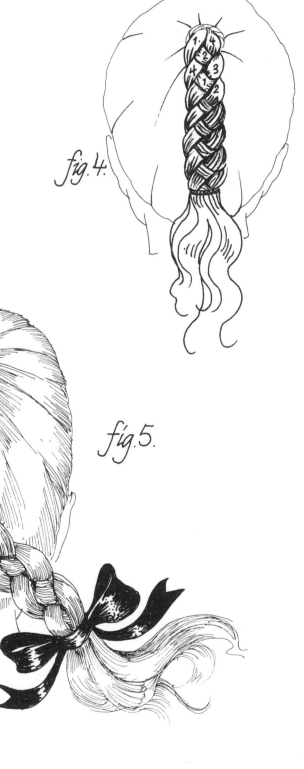

fig. 4.

fig. 5.

THE FOUR STRAND

— Separate the hair into four sections.

— Hold two strands in the right hand and two in the left hand.

— Start with strand #4, taking it over #3 strand, then under #2 strand.

— Take #1 and go under #4.

— The right outside strand always goes over and then under. The left outside strand only goes under.

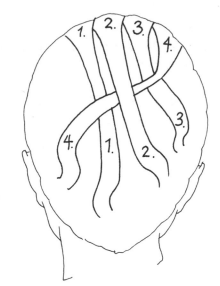

fig.1.

— Now feed into the braid every time the outside strand is picked up, both left and right.

— Take #3 strand and feed some hair into it.

— Cross over #2 and under #1.

— #4 goes under #3A.

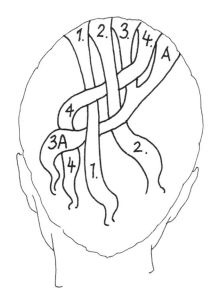

fig.2.

— Feed 'B' strand into #4, making it #4B.

— #4B goes under #3A.

— Return to the right side and repeat the feeding system, now using #2 on the right and #3A on the left.

— Remember to feed each outside strand before it travels.

— Figure 4 shows the completed four strand braid.

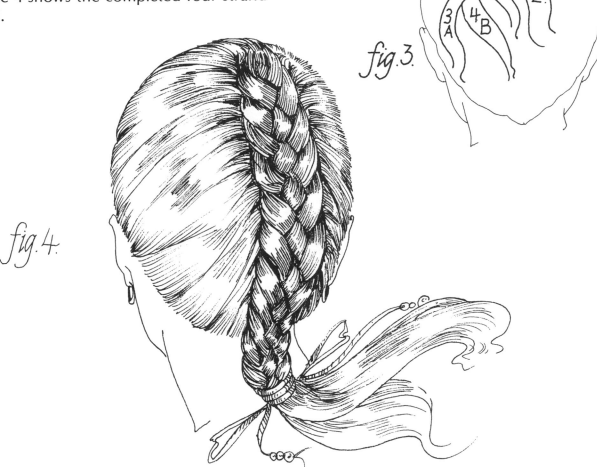

fig.3.

fig.4.

Helpful Hints

Hand Positions: Hold the strands equally, two left ones in the left hand, and two right ones in the right hand, for better control of braiding.

Adding-On: Hair must be added-on to both the right and left outside strands before they do any travelling.

FOUR STRAND
(Fed from Hairline only)

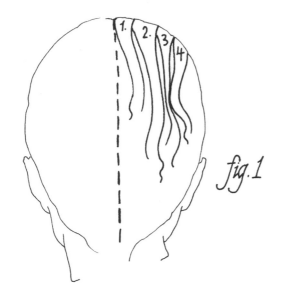

fig.1

— Make a center part (shown by the broken line).

— Divide hair on right side into four strands.

— Cross #4 over #3 and under #2.

— #1 goes under #4.

— Tighten strands.

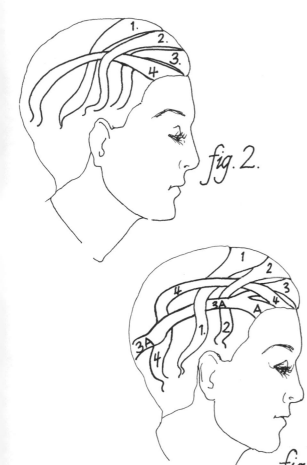

fig.2.

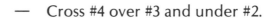
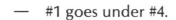

— Feed 'A' (pick up a new section of hair) into #3 strand.

— Take #3A, cross it over #2, under #1, then over #4.

— Repeat this step by going back to the hairline. Feed #2 this time, and take #2A over #1, under #4, and over #3A.

— Always feed the strand that is closest to the hairline, then go over, under, over.

fig. 3.

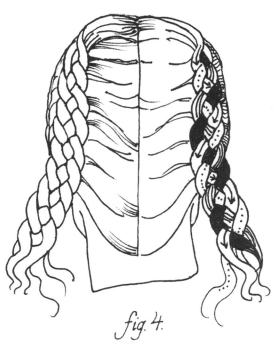

fig. 4.

— Continue this method until the right side is completed.

— Now do the braid on the left side, feeding only from the left hairline.

— Complete each side to the end of the pigtail, then fasten with an elastic.

— Figure 5 shows how the braids can be secured, the right braid under the left braid.

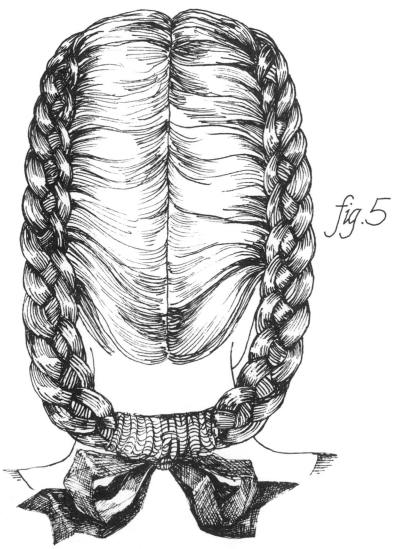

fig. 5

57

FOUR STRAND BRAID WITH CENTER PART

— The broken line represents a center part, from the front hairline to the back nape area.

— Take a triangular section on the right side of the part.

— Section it into four strands.

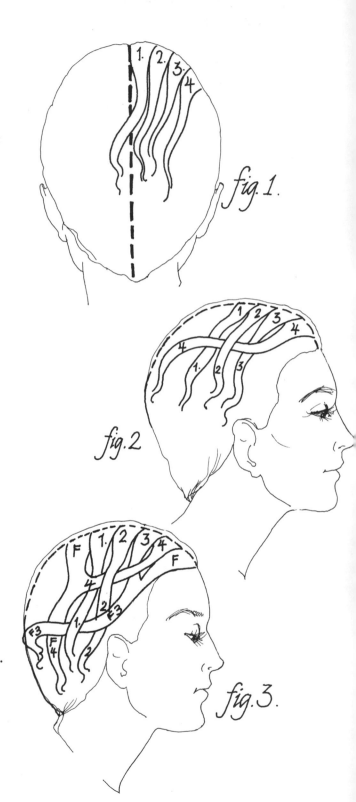

fig. 1.

— Cross #4 strand over #3, then under #2.

— #1 strand goes under #4.

fig. 2

— Feed some hair ('F') into #3.

— #3F crosses over #2 and under #1.

— Feed into #4. #4F goes under #3F.

— Continue braiding using this same method.

fig. 3.

— Remember when working on the right side of the head, this procedure is correct. On the left side, however, the procedure is slightly different.

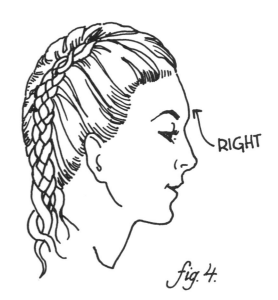

fig. 4.

— On the left side of the head, the outside strand (strand nearest the left ear) crosses over and then goes under.

— The outside strand nearest the center part goes under, always.

— Be sure to feed the outside strand after it has crossed over once.

— Continue in this manner until the braid is completed.

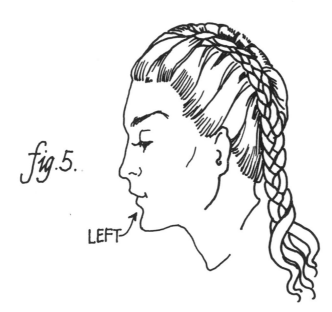

fig. 5.

LEFT

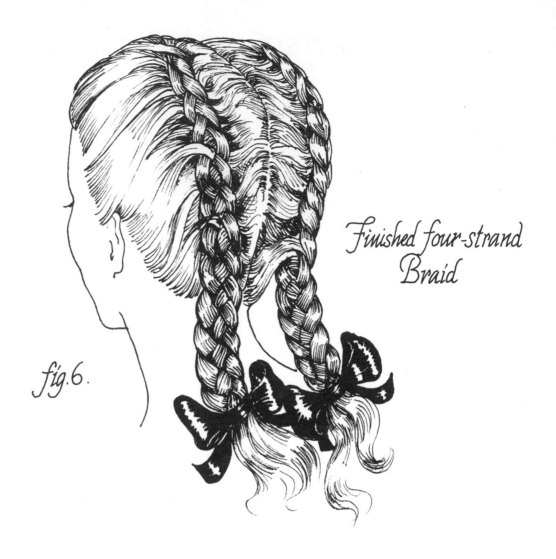

Finished four-strand Braid

fig.6.

Helpful Hints

Changing Sides: Braiding method reverses when moving from the right side to the left side. On the right side the right hand takes the strands over and under. When braiding the left side, the right hand only takes the strands under. This is important to remember since this braid will not finish properly otherwise.

FIVE STRAND PONYTAIL

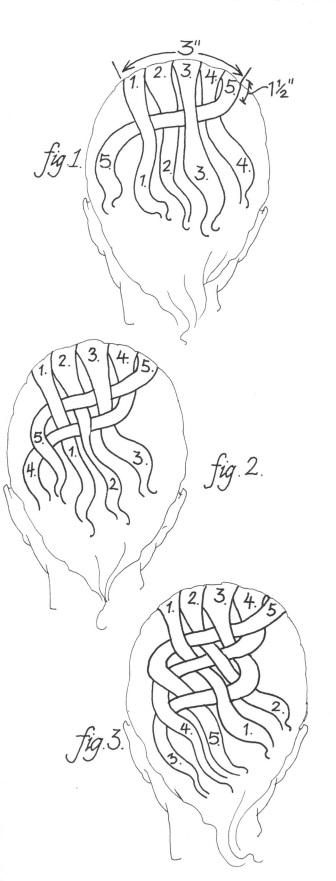

— Start at the forehead area.

— Make a horizontal section about 3" by 1½" and center it.

— Divide the section into five strands.

— Start at the right side of the section.

— Take strand #5, go over #4, under #3, over #2, and under #1.

— Start with the strands on the right, again on the outside.

— This time the outside strand will be #4. Take #4 and go over #3, under #2, over #1, and then under #5.

— Use strand #3 and go over #2, under #1, over #5, then under #4.

— Repeat this system until 2" to 3" from the end of the hair shaft.

— Tie off with an elastic.

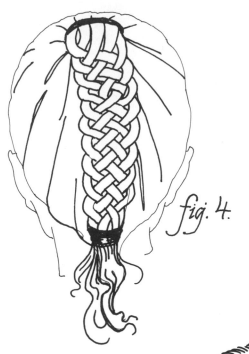

fig. 4.

— A completed five strand ponytail should resemble Figure 4.

— This ponytail is shown with loose tension only to show how the strands cross and go under one another.

— Figure 5 shows a five strand ponytail with tight tension.

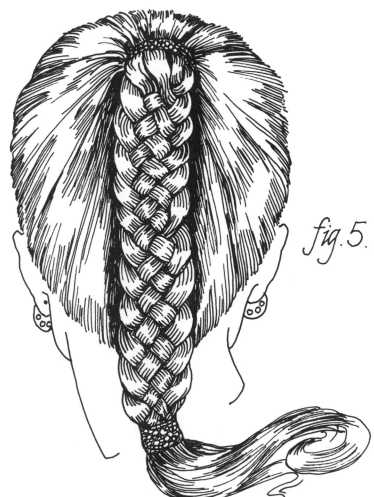

fig. 5.

6. *Fun With Braiding*

THE SNAKE COIL

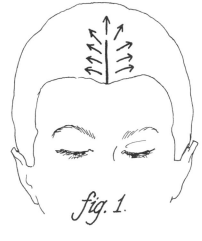

fig. 1.

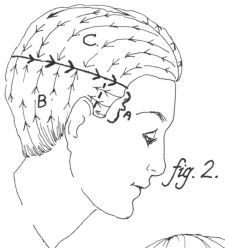

fig. 2.

— The solid line shows a part ending at the top center of the head. Arrows indicate the direction of hair to be smoothed down. The hair should lay flat and next to the head.

— Use the Invisible Braid method for this style. Start at the temple area in front of the ear, shown by the the dotted lines.

— 'A' arrows show three sections taken horizontally to begin the braid.

— 'B' arrows show the direction in which to feed into the braid from the bottom.

— 'C' arrows show the direction to feed from the top.

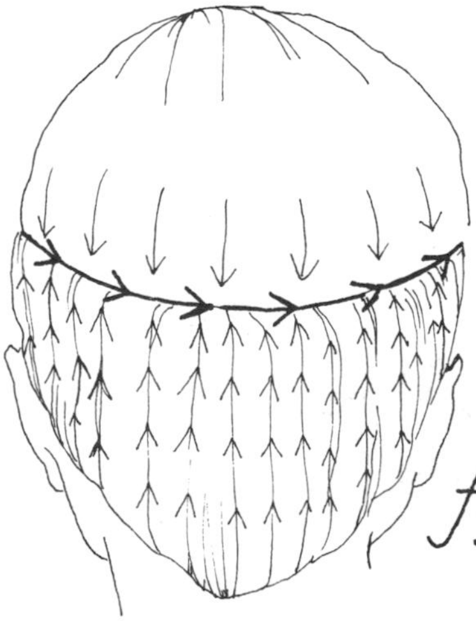

— Begin the braid one inch above the left ear. The braid goes horizontally around the head.

fig. 3.

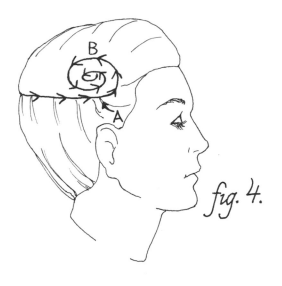

fig. 4.

- The braid is fed only until the front of the right ear is reached.

- Direct the hair in section 'A' back as one strand. Feed it into the braid.

- Complete the braid by making a pigtail.

- Place elastic on the end of the braid.

- Coil the braid as shown in 'B'.

- Secure the coil with bobby pins.

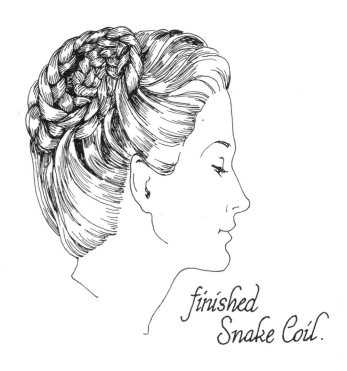

finished
Snake Coil.

DIAGONAL VISIBLE BRAID

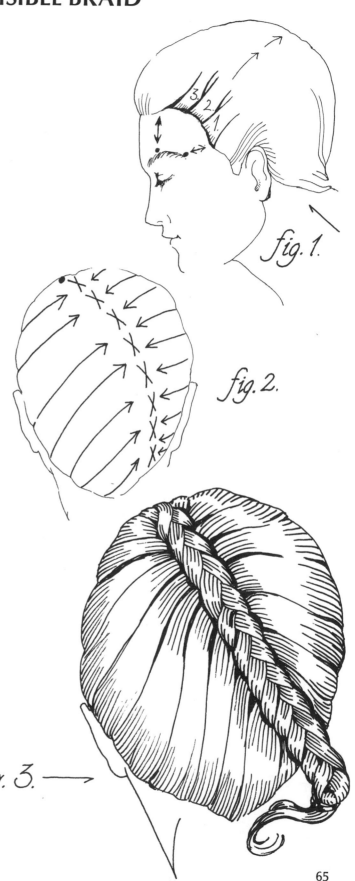

— When starting the braid section, strand #1 must be even with the end of the left eyebrow. Strand #2 should be even with the arch in the eyebrow. Strand #3 is even with the beginning of the left eyebrow.

— These arrows indicate the direction of the braid.

fig. 1.

fig. 2.

— The 'X's on Figure 2 symbolize the Visible Braid method. The braid should travel across the head in the same line as the 'X's. The arrows show that the hair is fed from the bottom and top, coming from the hairline on the left and the hairline on the right.

— The finished product looks as though the braid lays across the head. It is different from the Invisible Braid because the entire braid can be seen on top of the hair. (The plait cannot be seen when the Invisible Braid is worked.)

fig. 3. →

THE FISHTAIL

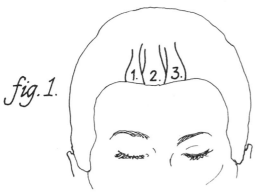

fig. 1.

— Start at the center front taking a small section of hair, and dividing it into three equal strands.

— Do an Invisible French Braid down the center of the head (from the forehead to the nape area).

— Continue braiding until pigtail section is finished.

— Hold the end of the tail braid in the left hand.

— With the right hand, fingers close together and thumb under fingers, work your way up to the crown area (marked 'X'). You'll be going up under the braid.

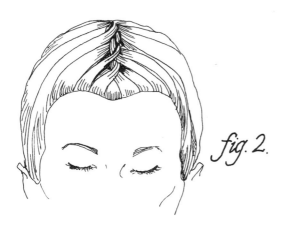

fig. 2.

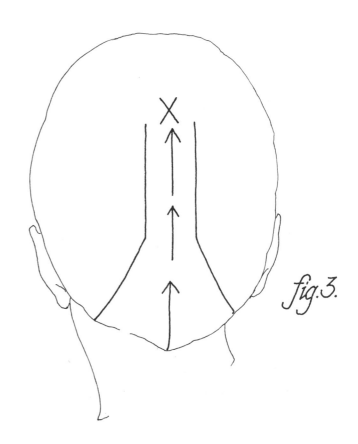

fig. 3.

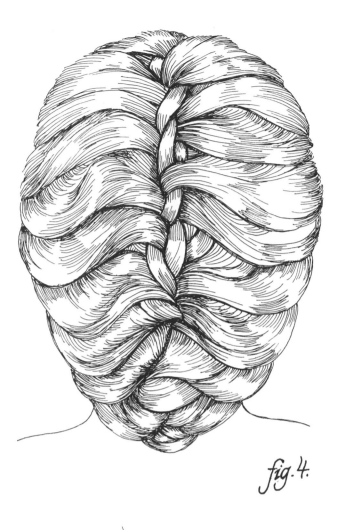

- Spread your right hand fingers out.

- Lift your hand up, away from the scalp.

- Shake your hand from left to right, moving it down toward the nape area.

- Finish braiding to the end of the tail and put a cloth covered elastic on.

- Tuck the braid underneath the fishtail and secure with a barrette. The barrette should pick up a bit of hair on the right side of the tail, then some more hair from the left of the tail before being fastened.

fig. 4.

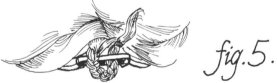

fig. 5.

- Figure 5 is an illustration of how the barrette should be fastened.

Helpful Hints

Barrette: Use a barrette that is all one piece, has no hinges, and is made of metal. Always fasten the barrette just underneath the elastic.

Even Fins: When lifting the hair away from the scalp, lift evenly to ensure that all fins on both sides of the head are the same length.

Finishing: Personal preference may be to leave the tail hanging loose.

THE REVERSE INVISIBLE BRAID

With the Reverse Invisible Braid, the plait begins at the nape. A bowed head is also necessary so that the braider can easily work with the nape area hair. Here again, the braider should stand directly in front of the person whose hair is being worked on.

The diagrams are shown upside down - as the person you'll be braiding will be in a bent over position. Have your lady sit in a chair, facing you, then have her bow her head.

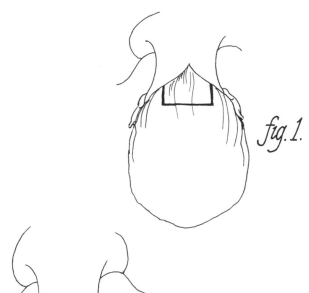

— Figure 1 shows the nape area. Take a section and the amount of hair shown.

— Divide the section into three equal strands.

— Cross strand #3 over strand #2.

— Take strand #1 over strand #3.

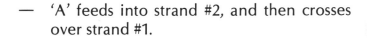

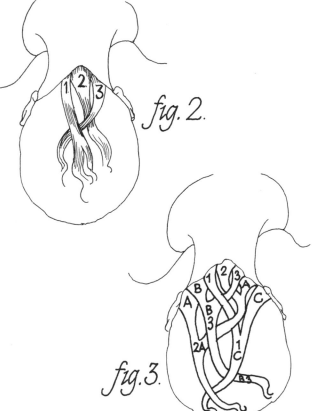

— 'A' feeds into strand #2, and then crosses over strand #1.

— 'B' feeds into strand #3, and crosses over strand #2A.

— Feed into #1 to make #1C.

— Feed into #2A and cross it over #1C.

— Continue this procedure to the crown area.

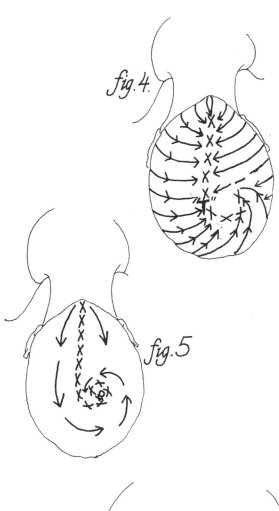

fig. 4.

fig. 5

— The lines with arrows represent feeding into the braid, and the direction the hair is taken.

— 'X' represents the braid. Braid Invisibly upward on the head.

— Note the 'T' formation in Figure 4. Start to feed from the hairline on the left only. The strand from the right will still cross over the center strand, but will not be fed. Direct the braid towards the right, as the 'X's show.

— After the last feed, continue the pigtail until two inches before the end and fasten with an elastic.

— Figure 5 shows how to put the pigtail in a circle. The 'O' in the drawing represents the elastic on the pigtail. Any hair at the end gets tucked under.

— Secure the coiled braid with a few bobby pins.

— The finished braid should resemble Figure 6.

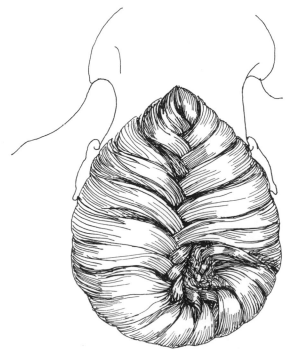

fig. 6.

THE GILLIAN BRAID

— The Gillian Braid is started with the same method as the Visible Braid.

— Strand #3 goes under #2.

— #1 goes under #3.

— When feeding, take sections that are only 1½" from the hairline toward the braid and 1" in width. The hair is picked up at the hairline, lays across other hair, and is then braided into a vertical Visible Braid at the center of the head.

— The Gillian Braid requires a minimum of five feed-in's on both sides, the right and the left.

— 'S' on each side of the braid signifies where to stop feeding. Notice the angle at which the last strand is fed in on the right and left sides.

— From this point braid one more turn, taking the hair directly underneath the braid.

— Do a Basic Braid (without feeding) for four more turns.

— Fasten with an elastic.

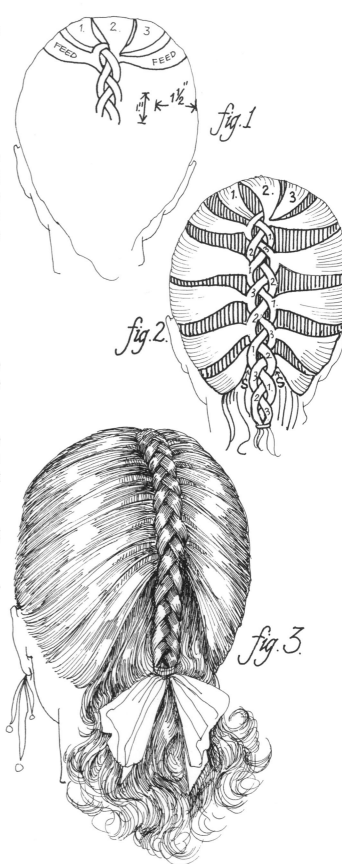

fig.1

fig.2

fig.3

70

THE JENNIFER BRAID

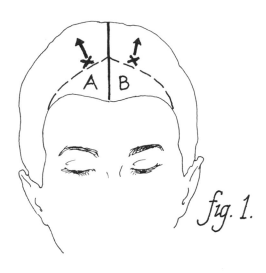

fig. 1.

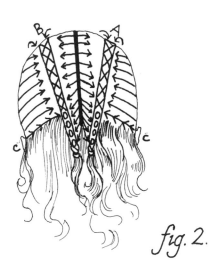

fig. 2.

— Make a center part (solid line).

— Part off sections 'A' and 'B' (broken lines).

— The center of each braid will be at 'X'.

— Arrows indicate the direction in which the braid will travel.

— 'X's indicate an Invisible Braid.

— Arrows show that the braid is fed from the center part and the hairline.

— 'O's represent feeding from the center part only.

— The arrows, marked 'C' indicate the last feed from the hairline, just behind the ear.

— Start with the left side.

— Make an Invisible Braid to the back of the ear.

— Now feed from the center part only and braid four turns.

— Braid another four turns (one turn equals right over and left over) without feeding.

— Secure with an elastic.

— The right side of the head is done with the same method.

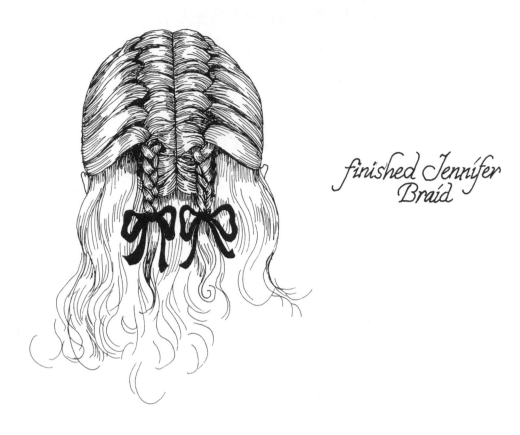

finished Jennifer
Braid

Helpful Hints

Line: Remember that the line of the braid should lie an inch from the center part.

THE CHEROKEE

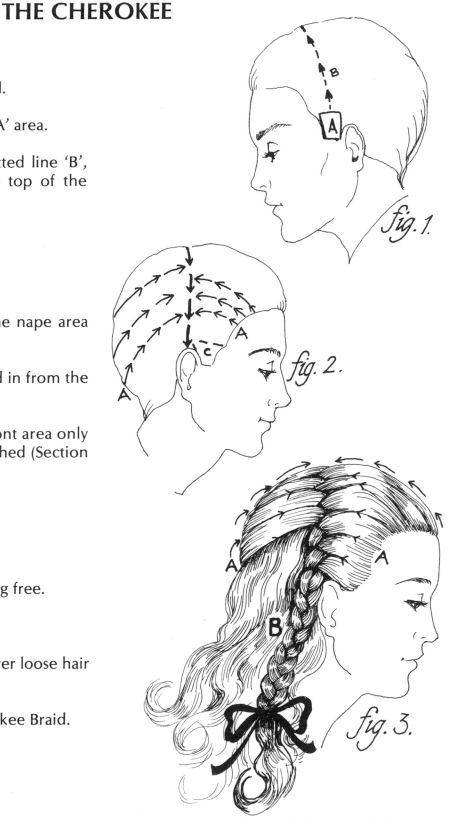

— Use the Invisible Braid method.

— Take a rectangular section at 'A' area.

— The braid is made on the dotted line 'B', going toward and across the top of the head.

— Arrows show feeding from the nape area and from the front hairline.

— Line 'A' is the last time to feed in from the back.

— Continue to feed from the front area only until the top of the ear is reached (Section 'C').

— The hair in section 'B' will hang free.

— It may hang straight or curled.

— Notice that the braid hangs over loose hair when finished.

— Figure 3 is a completed Cherokee Braid.

fig. 1.

fig. 2.

fig. 3.

Helpful Hints

Stance: Stand on the side opposite to which you are starting; stand where the braid will finish.

ANDRÉA'S CROWN BRAID

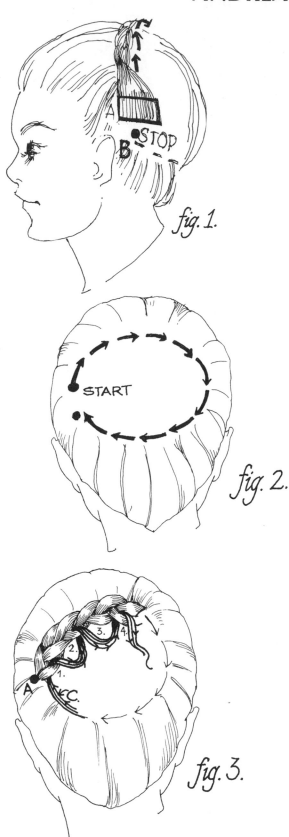

fig. 1.

fig. 2.

fig. 3.

— Begin at 'A'.

— Make a section 2 inches above the ear.

— Use the Modified Braiding method.

— Feed only from the hairline, all the way around the head to 'B'.

— Complete the braid by making a tail.

— Secure with an elastic.

— Tuck the end of the braid under the first section of the braid, at 'A'.

— Secure with bobby pins.

— If the hair is extremely long, the pigtail will be quite long.

— Take the end of the pigtail and loop it under and over #1, following arrow 'C'.

— Omit loop #2.

— Loop the end under and over #3, following arrow 'C'.

— Continue to loop the end in this manner until the whole pigtail is woven in.

— Tuck the elastic end under the braid. Secure the braid with bobby pins.

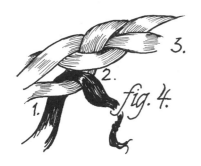

fig. 4.

— Figure 4 shows the crown section being looped with the pigtail.

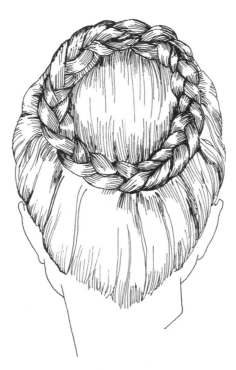

— See the color photo of the finished Crown Braid in the Photography Section.

THE COBRA

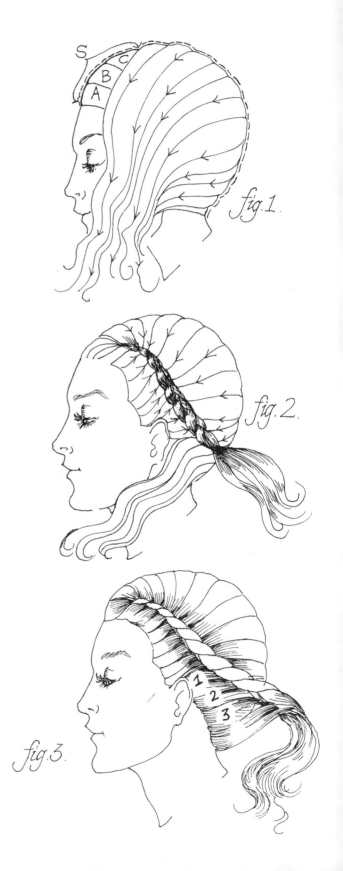

— Make a center part from the forehead to the nape.

— Take a pie shaped section from the hairline to the center part as 'S' indicates in Figure 1.

— The broken line is the part line.

— 'A', 'B', and 'C' are the three lines you'll be braiding with.

— The arrows going from the part to the hairline show the direction in which to comb the hair.

— Use the Invisible Braid method, feeding only from the hairline.

— Be aware of the direction you braid, as the braid should travel down the side of the head.

— Keep tight tension.

— When reaching #1 lift the hair away from head an inch. #2 feed will lift 1¼″, #3 1½″, and #4 2″, until all hair is fed in.

— Finish braiding the hair into a pigtail then fasten with an elastic.

fig.1.

fig.2.

fig.3.

— Figure 4 shows a front angle pose which illustrates how the braid hangs from the head (tight above the ear, looser below).

— Loop the braid, making a clockwise circle.

— Fold the elastic section of braid up and to the left so it lays on the circle formed by the braid. Fasten with a barrette, covering the majority of the elastic.

— A bow could also be used to fasten the tail, instead of a barrette.

— Figure 6 is a completed braid.

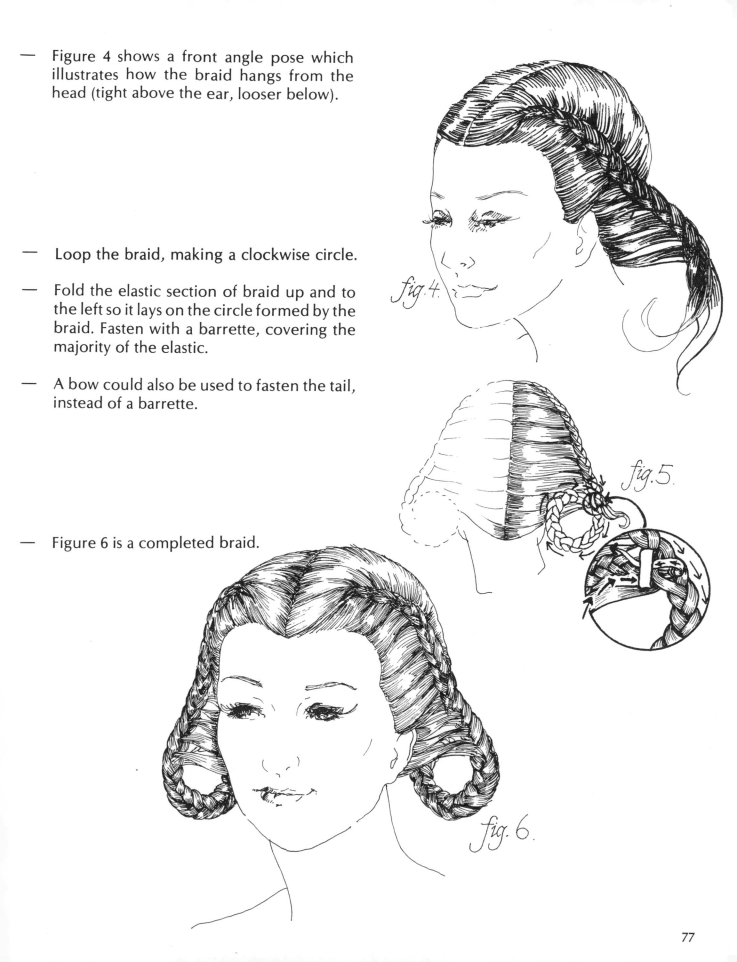

fig. 4.

fig. 5.

fig. 6.

THE VICKIE BRAID

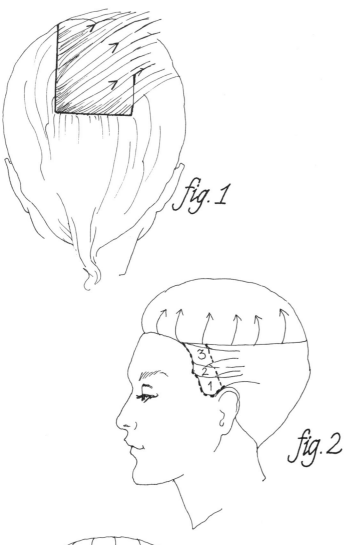

fig. 1

— Figure 1 shows how to part the hair," ⌐ " shape. Notice that the parted off section is placed to the right as shown by the arrows. This hair will be used later.

fig. 2

— The arrows going up designate the section clipped out of the way.

— Take a vertical section at the area shown by the broken lines.

— Work horizontally around the head, using the Invisible Braid method.

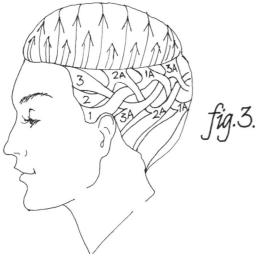

fig. 3.

— Figure 3 shows the Invisible Braid going horizontally around the head. (Drawn loosely only to show method.)

— Since feeding will be from both sides, allow enough room away from the part area to be able to pick up hair just beneath the part to feed into the braid.

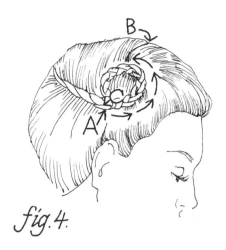

fig. 4.

— When point 'A' is reached, begin feeding from the bottom only (that is from the hairline and up).

— Release the clipped off section of hair so that it now hangs down, across the right ear and over part of the right side of the face. The three arrows show the direction the braid should be going.

— The 'B' area will be the last section of hair to be fed in.

— Finish the braid, like a pigtail, and tuck it under as in area 'C'.

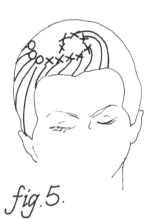

fig. 5.

— The 'O's represent the Invisible Braid.

— The 'X's represent the braid which is fed from the bottom only.

— Notice the slant of the lines. It is this angle that gives the "Vickie Braid" its special style. Be sure feeding has the angle or slant.

— Use pins to fasten the braid in place.

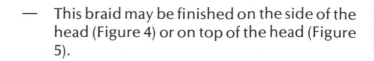

— This braid may be finished on the side of the head (Figure 4) or on top of the head (Figure 5).

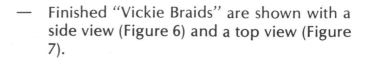

— Finished "Vickie Braids" are shown with a side view (Figure 6) and a top view (Figure 7).

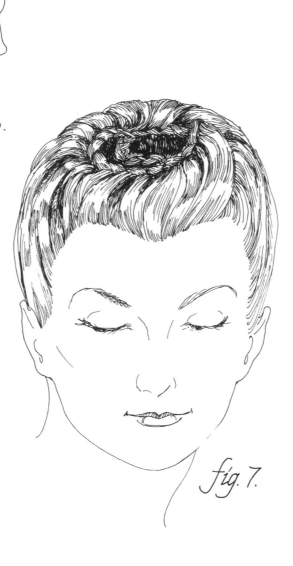

fig.6.

fig.7.

Helpful Hints

Finishing: With a long tail, coil the braid into place, then secure with pins.

THE TWIST BRAID

— Make a center part as indicated by the solid line. Notice that the part only goes ½" past the top of the center.

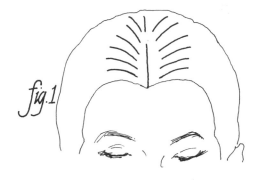

fig.1

— Divide the hair into two sections. The dotted line shows the center part. The hair will be hanging down from the part. Take #2 up and over #1.

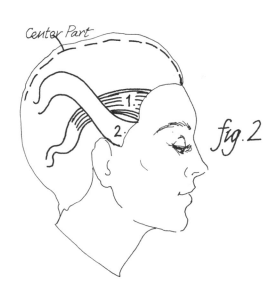

fig.2

Center Part

— Strand #2 comes down under #1, then up again over #1. #1 should now be hanging down.

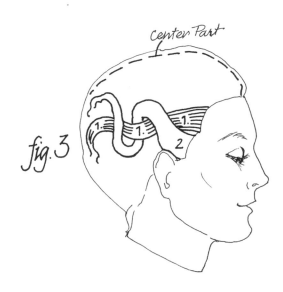

Center Part

fig.3

— #1 is fed from 'A' (bottom hair comes up from the hairline) and becomes #1A.

— #1A goes up and crosses over #2. #2 comes down.

— #2 is fed by 'A', and becomes #2A.

— #2A goes up and crosses over #1A.

— #1A comes down and is fed again.

— This procedure is repeated until the last section (in front of the left ear) is taken.

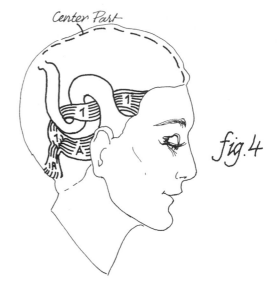

fig.4

— Continue twisting the two strands in the same direction, counter-clockwise around each other.

— Fasten with an elastic 1" to 2" from the end of the shaft.

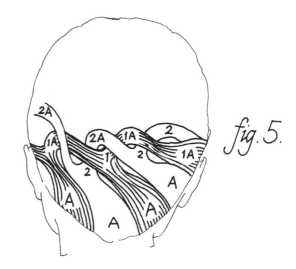

fig.5.

— 'S' is the last strand fed (opposite end of the twist tail).

— Start with 'S' area, wind (counter-clockwise). Twist tail up and around. See arrows for direction.

— Bring twist down and cross over 'S' section. Tuck the end of the tail into 'F' (Finish).

— Secure circular twist section with bobby pins.

— Figure 7 is the completed Twist Braid.

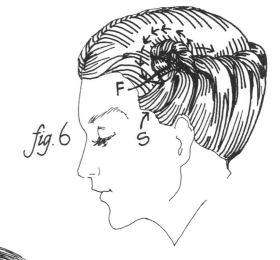

fig. 6

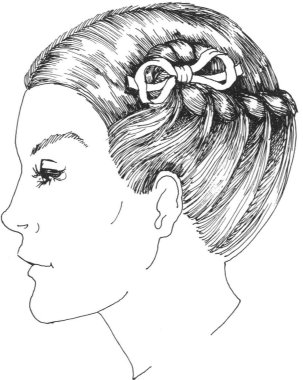

Helpful Hints

Feeding: One may also feed into the top strand if she finds that she has better control; consequently, having tighter tension. There will be a slight difference in the appearance of the braid.

THE RIBBON BRAID

Ribbon required: Very fine hair will need 1½ yards of ¼" width ribbon. Thick or heavy hair needs 1½ to 2 yards of ½" width.

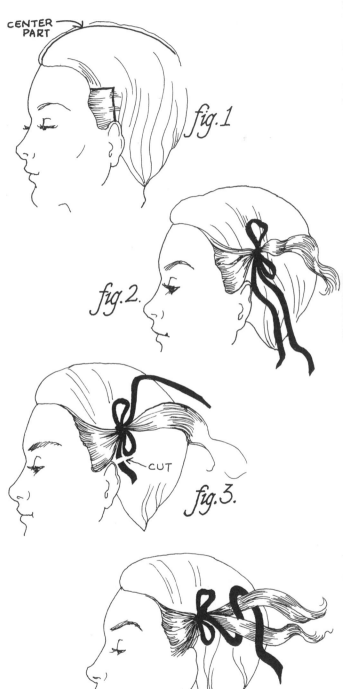

— Make a part from the center of the front hairline to two inches before the crown area. Comb the hair downward.

— Make a part at the temple area, as shown by the solid lines.

— Tie the ribbon in a bow around the hair section.

— Use eight inches of one end of the ribbon, the remainder will be used in braiding.

— Position the ribbon to start the braid. Only the long part of the ribbon is used in working the braid. The short end is cut off once the bow is tied.

— Divide the hair section into two strands, making the top strand thicker than the bottom strand.

— Take the ribbon under the bottom strand, up between the strands and over and around the top strand, down through the center and over the bottom strand.

— The ribbon will be hanging over the bottom strand (Figure 4).

— Take a strand of hair from the hairline and feed it into the bottom strand. Take the ribbon over and around the bottom strand, up through the center, over and around the top strand, down through the center again, and then hang it over the bottom strand.

— 'A' area shows the feeding of hair into the bottom strand. Repeat this procedure.

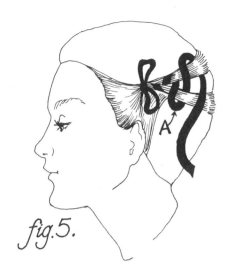

fig.5.

— The dark sections are ribbon.

— Continue weaving in and out between the two strands until the end of the hair is reached.

— Put an elastic on the end to secure the ribbon and hair tightly.

— The braid is shown across the top of the head, but it may also be put in a circle at the side, if desired. Use your imagination.

— Always secure the braid with bobby pins once its final position has been decided.

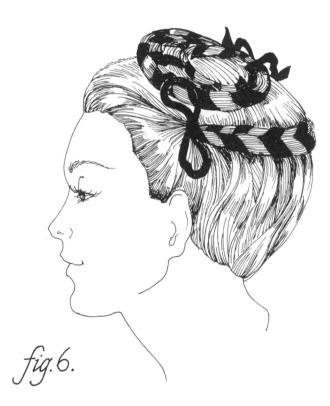

fig.6.

Helpful Hints

Ribbon Type: Gros-grain half-inch ribbon is recommended for long thick hair. Satin ribbon is too slippery to hold the hair well.

Variations: Use a side part instead of the center part, then finish the tail in a coil on the finishing side.

Weaving: If the top strand becomes too short add a strand of hair from above that section.

7. Variations of Ponytails and Pigtails

PONYTAIL KNOT

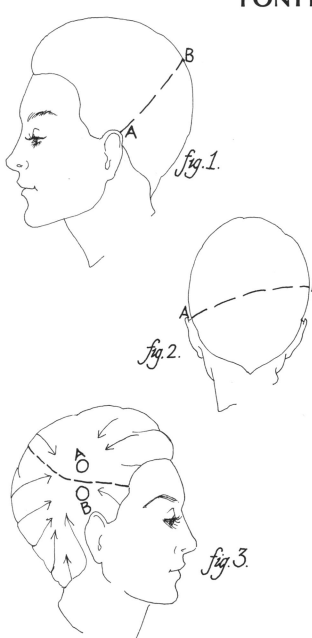

fig. 1.

fig. 2.

fig. 3.

— Start at 'A' and part hair from the top back of the ear to 'B', below the crown of the head.

— The back view of the part is 'A' to 'B'. It helps to see all three views of this style to get the pony tails into correct position.

— The dotted line is the part on the right side.

— 'A' designates where to secure the ponytail for the top area.

— 'B' shows where to secure the ponytail for the bottom area.

— Arrows indicate the direction in which to bring the hair from the hairline inward, to the ponytails.

— 'O' represents placement of the ponytails.

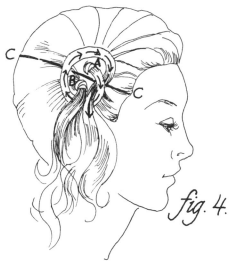

fig. 4.

— 'C' is a part between ponytails 'A' and 'B'.

— 'A', the top ponytail, does all the travelling.

— 'A' goes under 'B', up and over tied 'A' base; under 'A' strand (near the top) and out of the circle. Pull on the shaft of 'A' ponytail to form a secure knot.

— Secure knot with bobby pins at North, South, East, and West areas.

— Figure 5 shows the completed knot, once the tension has been tightened.

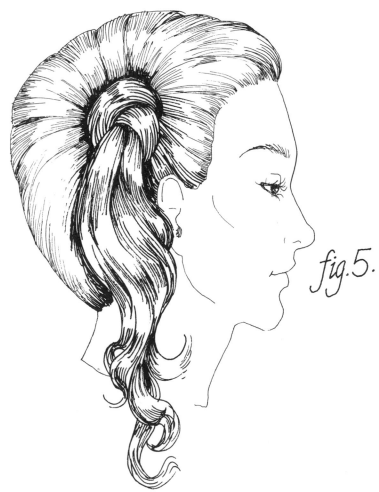

fig. 5.

FOUR PONYTAILS

— Part the hair as shown by the broken lines. Solid lines indicate where hair is brought down slightly so the part won't show.

— Bring the hair together to make ponytails at 'A', 'B', 'C', and 'D'.

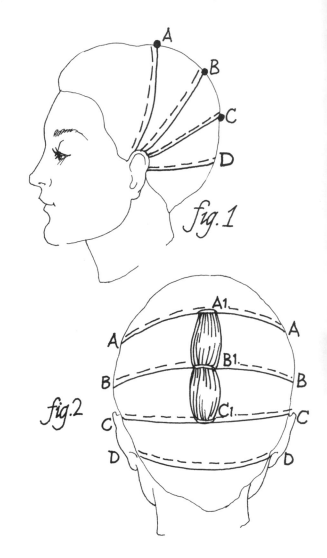

fig. 1

— 'A' goes completely across the head and is joined in a ponytail at A1.

— 'B' section stops on each side of the ponytail. The hair from 'B' is then joined with 'A' under the ponytail at B1.

— Do not pick up any hair under the ponytail.

fig.2

— Section 'C' is done the same way as 'B', including the ponytail which originally came from 'A'.

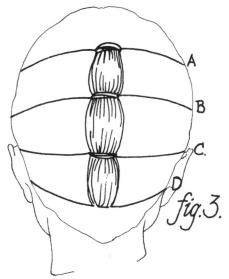

fig.3

— Do section 'D' in the same manner, this time bringing all remaining hair into the ponytail.

Variation:

— Start with section 1. Pull the hair on the outside of each section. (Spread the hair into a bulb shape.) Figure 5.

— Repeat, spreading sections 2 and 3.

— Colored elastics, or colored ribbon tied in bows, may be used to cover plain elastics.

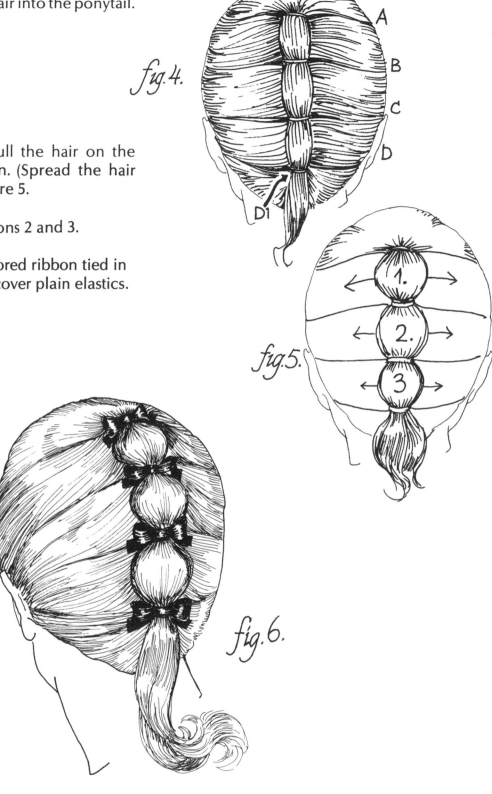

fig.4.

A

B

C

D

D1

fig.5.

1.

2.

3

fig.6.

THE GRECIAN

— The solid line is a center part from the
frontal hairline to the nape area.

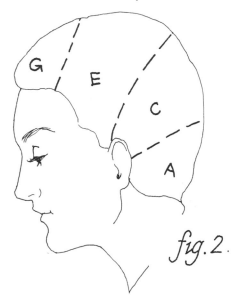

fig. 2.

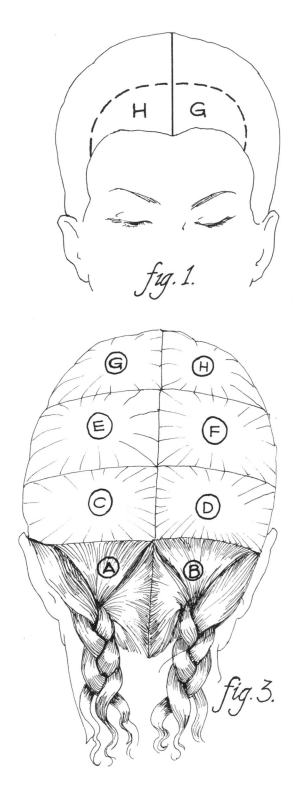

fig. 1.

— Figures 1, 2, and 3 show how the head is
sectioned into eight sections.

— Tie off each section, 'A' to 'H', individually.

— Each circled letter represents a braid.

— Starting with section 'A', braid a regular
pigtail.

— Hold the hair toward the bottom of the
section as the hair is braided down.

— The base of the braid should lay flat against
the head.

— Do not lift the base as you would in a
ponytail. (See Figure 3, Sections 'A' and 'B'.)

— Complete the braid to nearly the end and
secure with a small elastic.

— Braid all sections 'A' to 'H'.

fig. 3.

— Join the braids to one another.

— Start with 'A'. Put the end of 'A' under braid 'B'. (Be sure the elastic is under the base so it doesn't show.)

— Take a thin pipe cleaner and put it under some of the base hair, to the right of the pigtail, then under the elastic (keeping the elastic above the pipe cleaner) and then under some base hair to the left of the elastic.

— Bring the pipe cleaner ends together and fasten over the top of the pigtail.

— Twist the pipe cleaner ends together securely. (Be sure the pipe cleaner is far enough under 'B' base so it does not show.) The length of pipe cleaner used will be determined by the circumference of the pigtail.

— Follow the procedure in Figure 4 to put:
'B' under 'C'
'C' under 'F'
'D' under 'E'

— Continue this procedure as in Figure 5:
'F' under 'E'
'E' under 'F'
'G' under 'H'
'H' under 'G'

— Arrows indicate the direction the braid goes, from one base to another.

— As the braids are secured, they will overlap as they hang down.

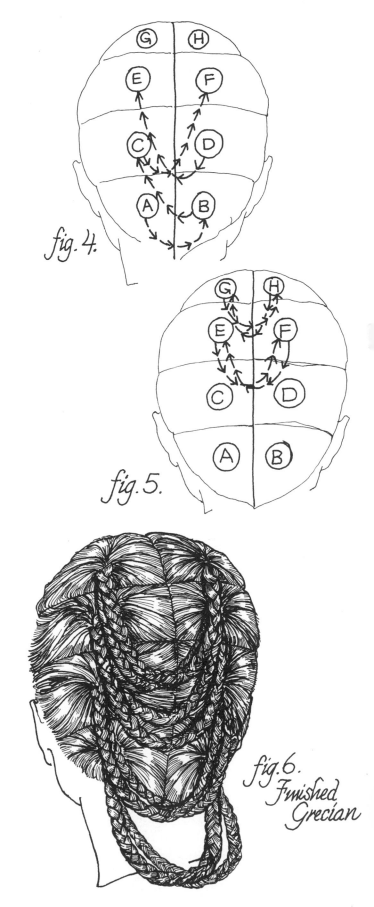

fig. 4.

fig. 5.

fig. 6.
Finished Grecian

Helpful Hints

Sectioning: Sectioning can be done all at once, before any braiding is done, or as needed so long as the sections remain even.

Very Long or Thick Hair: Do more sections as thinner braids are easier to work with and can also be secured better.

8. Rolls

PONY ROLL

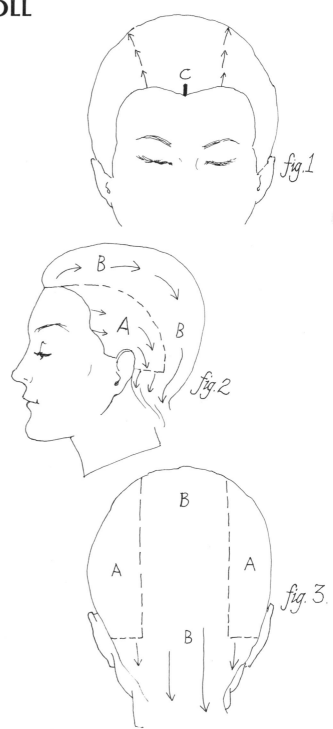

fig. 1

fig. 2

fig. 3

— 'C', with the solid line, symbolizes the center at the frontal area.

— Make a part, 1" from the center on both sides. Follow the direction of the arrows, from the forehead hairline, down the back of the head.

— Figure 2 illustrates how to section the hair on the left side. The right side is sectioned in the same way.

— Follow the broken lines for proper sectioning.

— Figure 3 illustrates a back view of the sectioning.

— Section 'B' hangs down the back of the head.

— Bring both 'A' sections together.

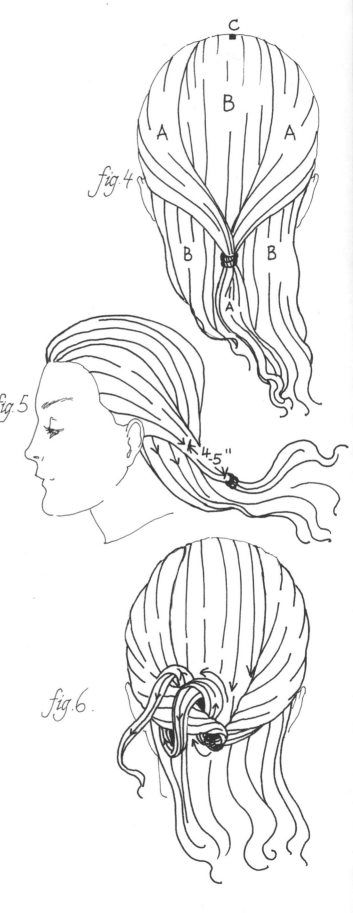

— Join the 'A' sections.

— Notice the angle at which the 'A' sections are directed and held (45°).

fig. 4

— Hold 'A' sections four to five inches away from and below the occipital bone, as indicated in Figure 5.

— Fasten with an elastic.

fig. 5

— Lift the ponytail up and put it down through the top as shown in Figure 6.

— The elastic section goes a full circle around, ending up where it began.

fig. 6.

— To achieve the same effect as Figure 7, one
   must loop the ponytail around and through
   the top section twice.

— For every loop the result will be more roll
   on the sides.

— Figure 7 is completed Pony Roll.

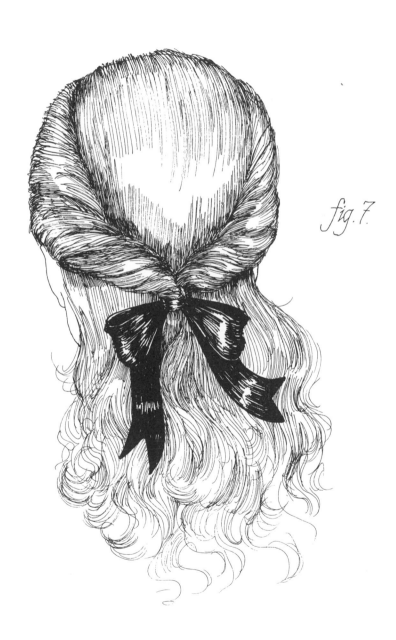

fig. 7

THE HALF TIE ROLL

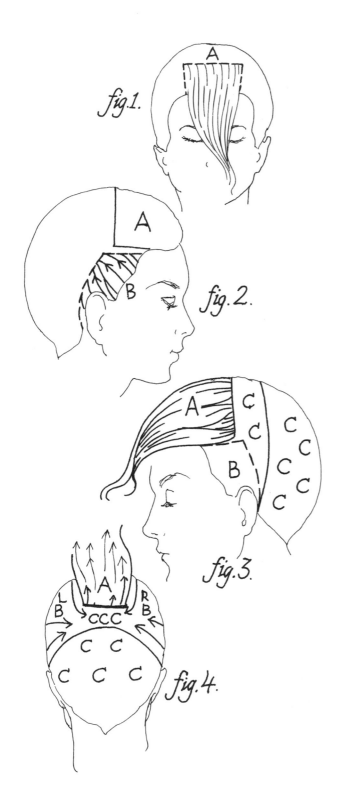

fig. 1.

fig. 2.

fig. 3.

fig. 4.

— Section the hair along the dotted line.

— Comb the section forward and clip or put in an elastic for now. This section will be used later in Figure 7.

— Make section 'B', as shown by the dotted line.

— Bring section 'B' to the crown area, just below section 'A'.

— Comb up at an angle (see arrows).

— Do not take any hair from 'C' area. 'B' area (from both the left and right sides) will be brought over area 'C'.

— Section 'B' comes directly under 'A', and over the top of 'C'.

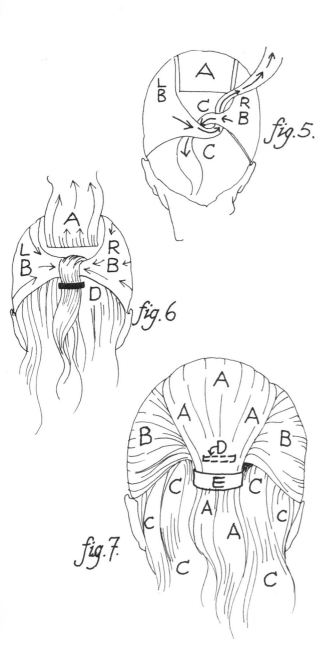

— Tie left 'B' and right 'B', as shown.

— Bring the shaft of 'LB' back over 'RB'. Join together with a clasp, 'D'.

— Bring section 'A' over section 'B' and clasp 'D'.

— Tie clasp 'E' around section 'A' (just below 'D' clasp).

— Pick up some hair from 'C' section to include underneath clasp 'E'.

— The finished Half Tie Roll.

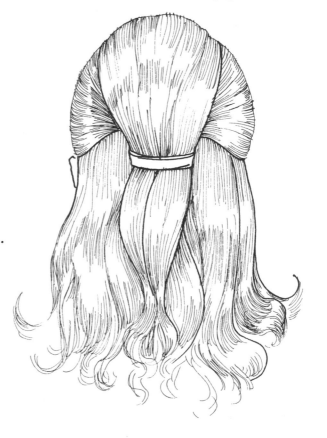

fig. 8.

THE FRENCH ROLL

— Bring hair up at a 45° angle. To 'lock' the roll in, place pins underneath the rolled hair.

— Pins should point upwards, towards the top of the head, not downward.

— Keep the roll even and centered.

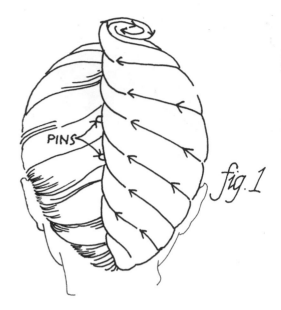

fig.1

— Put the shaft into a coil between the crown area and hairline at the forehead. Place the hair as shown by the arrows.

— Figure 3 illustrates a completed French Roll.

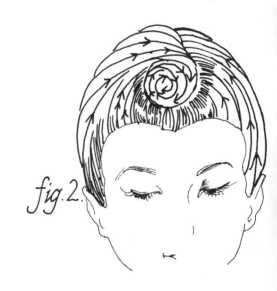

fig.2.

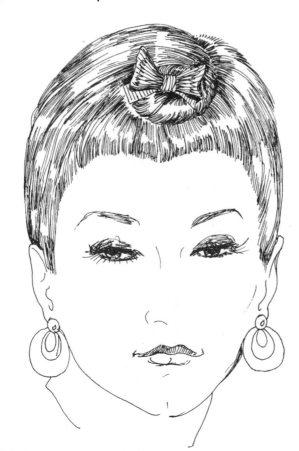

fig.3.

THE COMPLETE ROLL

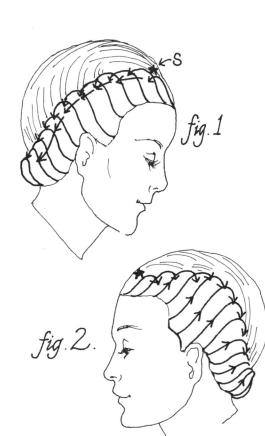

fig. 1

— Right side, start roll at 'S'.

— The roll flows along the double line.

— Place pins at the arrows.

— To do the left side, use the same procedure as on the right side.

fig. 2.

— The roll comes down from the top left and ends at 'F', just right of the center nape area.

— A finished Complete Roll.

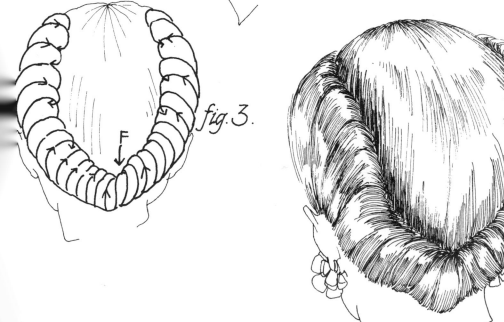

fig. 3.

fig. 4.

DIAGONAL ROLL

— Start at the nape area of the hairline, behind the left or right ear.

— Figure 2 shows the starting point, if starting at the right ear.

— Bring hair up from the nape area, rolling it under, a section at a time, 'A', 'B', 'C', and 'D'.

— Join the sections carefully so that there are no separations.

— The roll will start narrow, getting wider as it moves up the head.

— The roll travels around the head, on an angle, ending in a coil near the hairline.

— The completed Diagonal Roll.

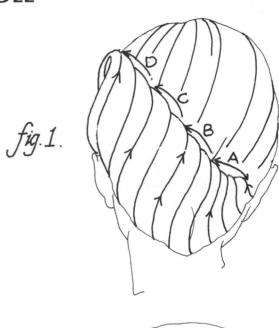

fig.1.

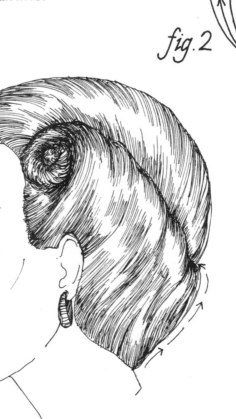

fig.2

START

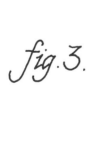

fig.3.

VERTICAL FRENCH ROLL WITH FLOWING NAPE

— Comb the hair straight down toward nape area.

— Section off the area marked with broken lines.

— Comb the hair in section 'A' downward.

— Comb the hair in section 'B' to the right.

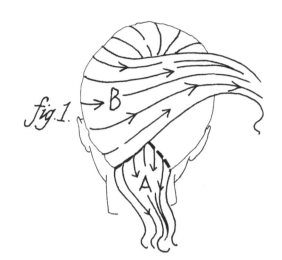

fig. 1.

— Arrows show the direction in which the hair is to be combed.

— Smooth the 'B' section.

— Place bobby pins, in an upward direction, along the middle as shown by the arrows.

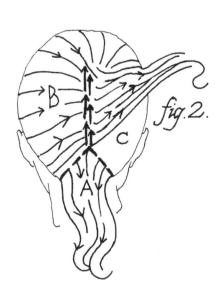

fig. 2.

— Now brush the hair from the right side towards the middle, and roll it under, securing with bobby pins. Place the pins downward vertically.

— Arrows proceeding down, left of the center, represent the bobby pins.

— Arrows in 'B' and 'C' sections designate the direction in which the hair should be brushed.

— Curl the hair in section 'A', which will be hanging loose.

— Figure 4 shows the completed hair style.

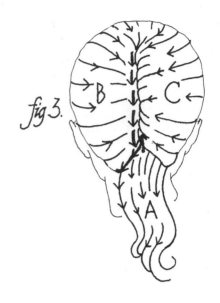

fig 3.

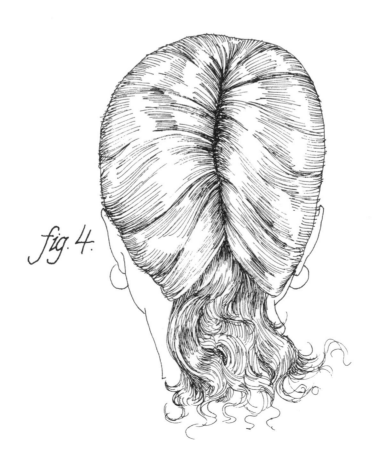

fig. 4.

CHIGNON

— Brush the hair in the direction shown by the arrows.

— The Chignon may be swirled clockwise or counter-clockwise.

— Place the index finger at 'A'.

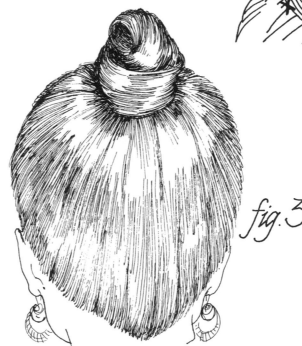

— Wrap the shaft of the strand around the index finger, placing bobby pins as shown by the 'X's in Figure 2.

— Continue around the index finger, working toward the top of the Chignon.

— Place the end of the hair shaft through the center (which is a hole) and secure with a bobby pin.

— The completed Chignon.

Helpful Hints

Placement: Chignons can be placed on the top of the head, at the back of the crown, or on either side of the head just above the temple.

TWISTED FIGURE-OF-EIGHT

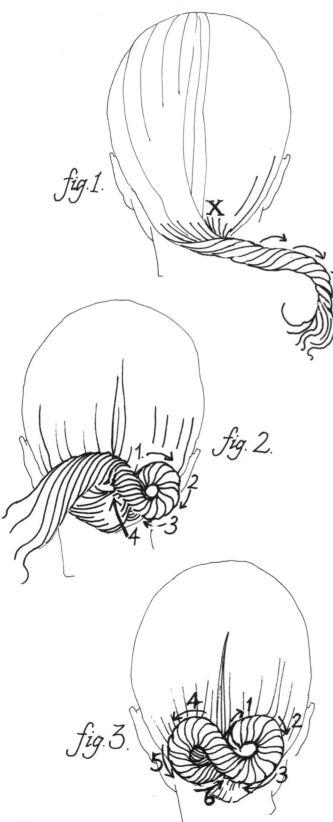

— Comb the hair into one strand straight down the back of the head.

— Bring the hair into one strand between the center of the nape area and the back right ear (at 'X').

— Twist the strand clockwise, making it as tight as possible.

— Numbered arrows indicate the direction to take the twisted strand.

— Complete the Figure-of-Eight by going from steps one to five.

— Secure the entire twist with bobby pins, placing some of the pins at areas 1, 2, 3, 4, and 5.

fig. 1.

fig. 2.

fig. 3.

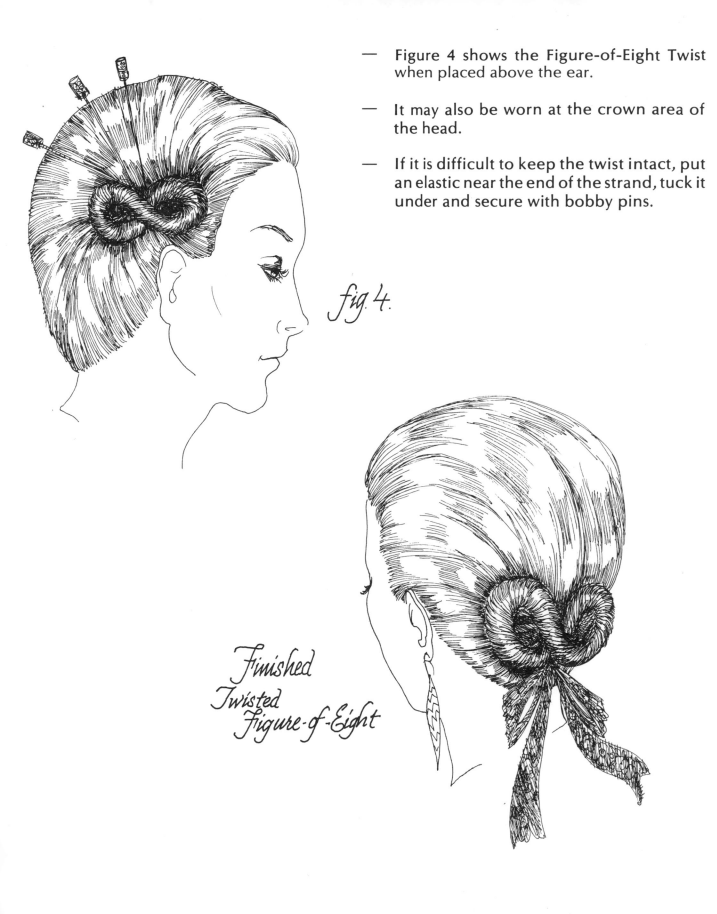

— Figure 4 shows the Figure-of-Eight Twist when placed above the ear.

— It may also be worn at the crown area of the head.

— If it is difficult to keep the twist intact, put an elastic near the end of the strand, tuck it under and secure with bobby pins.

fig. 4.

Finished Twisted Figure-of-Eight

NOTES:

NOTES:

NOTES:

Please send:

☐   Copies of BRAIDS & MORE

☐   Copies of BRAIDS & STYLES FOR LONG HAIR

        $19.95 per copy

_____ GST (7% of Book Total Balance for CANADA ONLY)

_____ $3.00 for POSTAGE & HANDLING IN CANADA

_____ $4.00 for POSTAGE & HANDLING IN U.S.A.

MAIL ALL ORDERS TO: **BRAIDS & STYLES FOR LONG HAIR**
        P.O. Box 73054
        #206, 2525 Woodview Drive S.W.
        Calgary, AB
        Canada T2W 6E4

CHEQUES AND MONEY ORDERS MADE PAYABLE TO, "BRAIDS & STYLES FOR LONG HAIR".

Name _____

Address _____

City _____ Province of State _____

Country _____ Postal Code or Zip Code _____

THANK YOU!

Please send:

☐   Copies of BRAIDS & MORE

☐   Copies of BRAIDS & STYLES FOR LONG HAIR

        $19.95 per copy

_____ GST (7% of Book Total Balance for CANADA ONLY)

_____ $3.00 for POSTAGE & HANDLING IN CANADA

_____ $4.00 for POSTAGE & HANDLING IN U.S.A.

MAIL ALL ORDERS TO: **BRAIDS & STYLES FOR LONG HAIR**
        P.O. Box 73054
        #206, 2525 Woodview Drive S.W.
        Calgary, AB
        Canada T2W 6E4

CHEQUES AND MONEY ORDERS MADE PAYABLE TO, "BRAIDS & STYLES FOR LONG HAIR".

Name _____

Address _____

City _____ Province of State _____

Country _____ Postal Code or Zip Code _____

THANK YOU!